Pedaling Through the Years

Other Books by the Author

A SERIOUS CYCLIST'S GUIDE
to SAN FRANCISCO and BEYOND
[2024]

EL RONDÍN
by Esteban Luján
Translated by Jonathan Van Coops
[2019]

Cover Image:
Climbing Monitor Pass in The World's Toughest Triathlon
[September 7, 1985]
by Thomas H. Mikkelsen

Pedaling Through the Years

Stories of a Cycling Life

By

Jonathan Van Coops

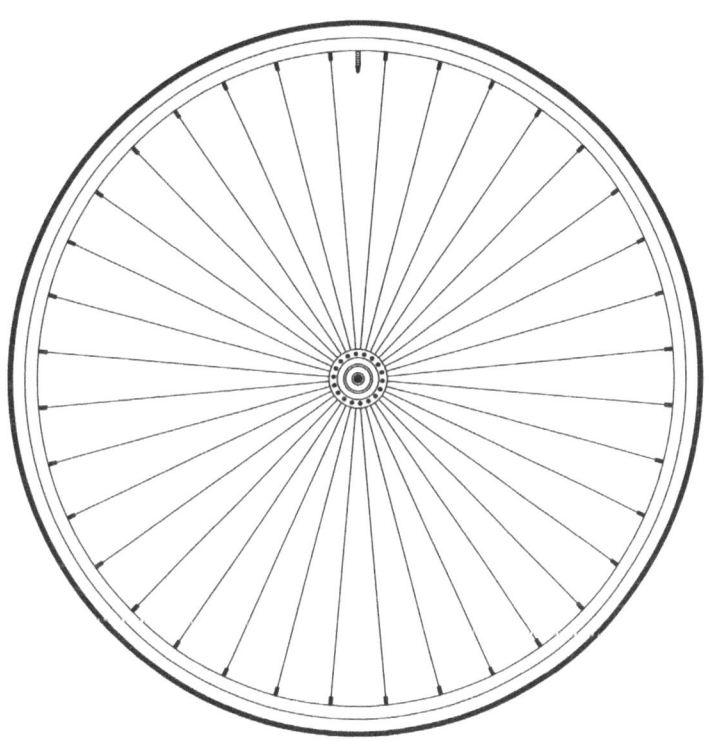

REGENT PRESS
Berkeley, California

©2025 by Jonathan Van Coops
[paperback]
ISBN 10: 1-58790-705-4
ISBN 13: 978-1-58790-705-0
[e-book]
ISBN 10: 1-58790-706-2
ISBN 13: 9-781-58790-706-7

Library of Congress Cataloging-in-Publication Data

Names: Van Coops, Jonathan, 1954- author
Title: Pedaling through the years : stories of a cycling life / By Jonathan Van Coops.
Description: Berkeley, California : Regent Press, [2025] | Includes index. | Summary: "Every serious cyclist accumulates stories about their riding adventures. With tales of the 'first' bike, cycling to the 1984 summer Olympics in Los Angeles, racing in the World's Toughest Triathlon, seeing the Tour de France first hand and more, Pedaling Through the Years is a lifelong cyclist's memoir, a collection of sixteen stories that illustrate cycling's blissful, funny or frightful moments and its unending potential for making unique two-wheeled experiences entertaining and unforgettable"-- Provided by publisher.
Identifiers: LCCN 2025021527 (print) | LCCN 2025021528 (ebook) | ISBN 9781587907050 trade paperback | ISBN 9781587907067 ebook
Subjects: LCSH: Van Coops, Jonathan, 1954- | Cyclists--California--Biography | Cycling--Anecdotes | LCGFT: Biographies
Classification: LCC GV1051.V325 A3 2025 (print) | LCC GV1051.V325 (ebook)
LC record available at https://lccn.loc.gov/2025021527
LC ebook record available at https://lccn.loc.gov/2025021528

All rights reserved. No part of this book may be used or reproduced in any manner whatsoever without written permission except in the case of brief quotations embodied in articles and reviews. For information, write to Jonathan Van Coops at jonvc321@gmail.com.

Photographs by Thomas H. Mikkelsen and Frank Varvaro are used by permission of the photographers, who retain sole copyright to them. ©2025
Sole copyright to images by the author is retained by Jonathan Van Coops. ©2025

Printed and bound in the United States of America
Regent Press
Berkeley, California
www.regentpress.net
email: regentpress@mindspring.com

Contents

Introduction

The First Bike (1963)   3

The Film of Sand (1964)   7

Slip Sliding Away: Oil on the Mountain (1983)   15

Those First Scratches! (1983)   21

Truckin' through Sausalito (1984)   29

Cycling to Los Angeles for the Summer Olympic Games (1984)   33

Chased Down and Dropped by the Swiss Olympic Team (1984)   49

Road and Track Cycling at the XXIII Olympiad (1984)   53

The *World's Toughest Triathlon* or Poppin' the Hip (1985)   59

Rolling a Sew-up (1990)   75

Hookin' Handlebars (1990)   83

Critical Mass (1992)   93

RAMROD – The Ride Around Mount Rainier in One Day (1993)   105

STP – Seattle to Portland (1994)   113

CRASH! The Great Highway Romp and Getting 'Doored' (1999)   127

My Very Own *'Tour de France'* (2006)   137

Index of Selected Places   201

Acknowledgements   203

About the Author   204

Introduction

Every serious cyclist accumulates stories about their riding adventures – I'm no exception. Maybe the exception is being able to write about those adventures, incidents *and accidents!* With tales of my first bike, cycling to the 1984 summer Olympics in Los Angeles, racing in the 1985 World's Toughest Triathlon, seeing the 2006 Tour de France firsthand and more, **Pedaling Through the Years** is part of a lifelong cyclist's memoir. It is a collection of sixteen stories that illustrate some of cycling's blissful, funny or frightful moments and its unending potential for making unique two wheeled experiences unforgettable. The stories also present an opportunity to acknowledge others who played a part in creating recollections that endure.

I grew up riding the streets and roads of San Francisco's East Bay area beginning in the early 1960s. I learned to ride in a day and have never stopped pedaling through the years. As an adult I became a serious cyclist – mostly a medium to long distance *road* cyclist. My riding friends and I covered a lot of ground throughout the last 40 years, becoming decent climbers by necessity and accumulating an array of cycling stories while continually training and completing various San Francisco area 'century' rides and west coast long distance cycling events.

In addition to being a lover of cycling, I'm a professional cartographer – a map maker and geographer – who had a long career involved in mapping California's Coastal Zone[*] before retiring in 2015. Since then, having not only time to ride but to *write*, I decided to produce a set of maps and cycling stories about some of my most memorable rides.

Pedaling Through the Years recounts some remarkable rides and riding. It's a chronicle of cycling adventures that I endeavored to present in a manner that encourages others to get out there and ride, to participate in creating their own premium cycling adventures and perhaps to record or write about experiences that become part of *their* cycling life. *Allez!*

Jonathan Van Coops   San Francisco, March 2025

---

* The Coastal Zone in California extends along the shore and includes adjacent inland areas in all coastal and San Francisco Bay Area counties.

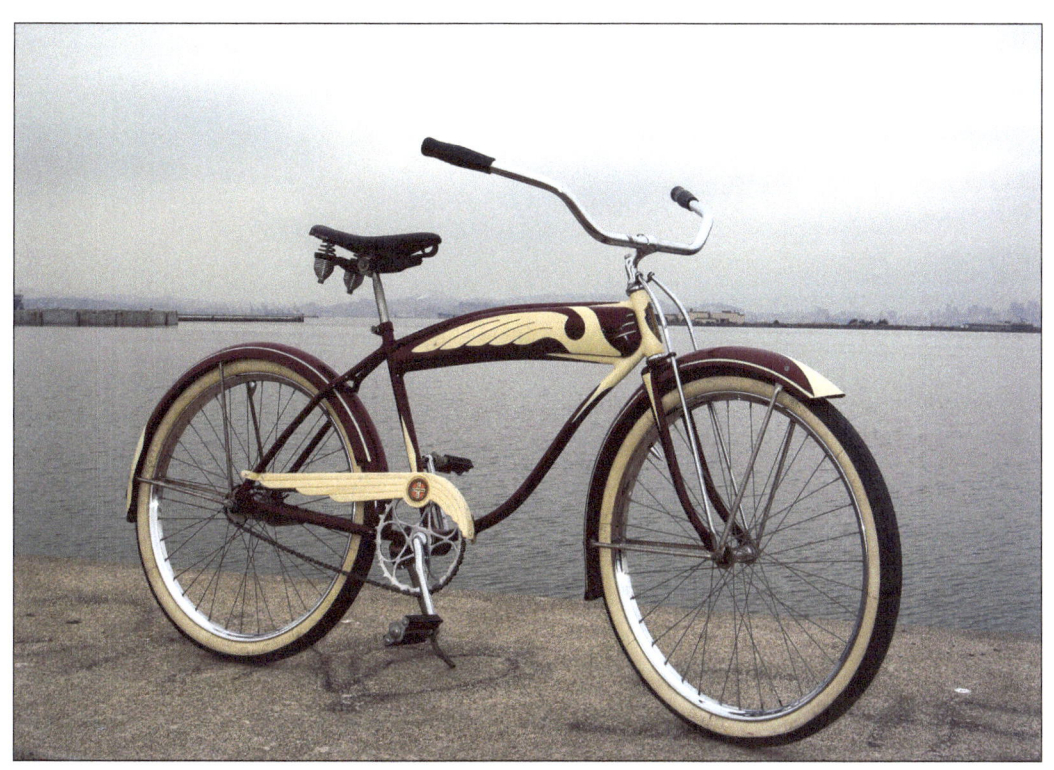

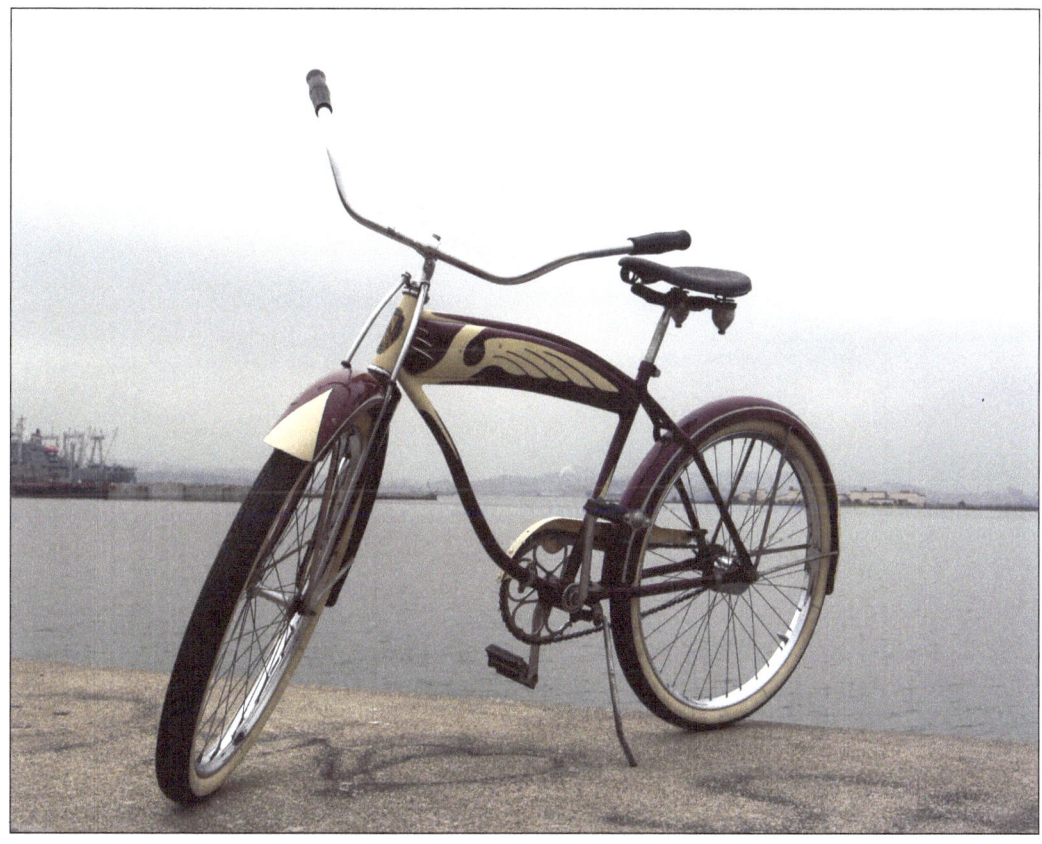

On San Francisco Bay with an all-time favorite – my 1939 Schwinn Century

I live the life I love... and I love the life I live
– WILLIE DIXON
  Legendary 20th Century American songwriter and blues guitarist

The First Bike (1963)

I was about eight years old when I taught myself how to ride a neighbor girl's bicycle. It was 1963, when my family was living in the Contra Costa County town of Pinole, California. The bike was a *Schwinn* with a 'girl's' frame – no top tube – what we might now call a 'step-through' design. With a single speed and 'coaster' brake, it was simple and solid. I'd watched it developing a rusty chain and nicely faded, chalky white paint – sunbaked on one side after several years of leaning untouched in the side yard against their garage.

I asked if I could borrow it one day and her surfboard-designing dad said 'okay.' Their family had moved to Pinole from southern California but I've never forgotten his cowboy drawl or the wisdom in his response – one for a serious cyclist's quote book:

"You be careful and jus' remember… you can 'git goin' *awful fast* on a one speed bike."

At the time, it sounded more like a joke than something ominous. My sense of imminent fun had me oblivious to how this adage *"awful fast"* might eventually play out in my cycling life. I would become only too aware later on, repeatedly, but right then I was grinning from ear to ear – I had a bike to ride! I rolled it into our garage, cleaned and oiled the chain as best I could and used my brother's basketball pump to inflate the tires.

The bike was much too small for me but so easy to balance on its twenty inch wheels. I couldn't fall down. Before long I had raised the seat as far as possible and reversed the direction of the handlebars, giving the front of the bike a sort of 'cattle horn' look, similar to track racing bikes of the 1980s and modern 'road' handlebars with upturned brake lever hoods. I had no idea I was channeling a future standard – I just needed to extend my reach and knee clearance enough to make *'Whitey'* rideable.[1] I had nothing but fun with this bike! There was nothing to fear. It made no difference whether or not the fit was correct. I was tall for my age and skinny. The bike was small and easy to maneuver.

---
1. Many of the bikes I've owned over the years have been 'named' for their color.

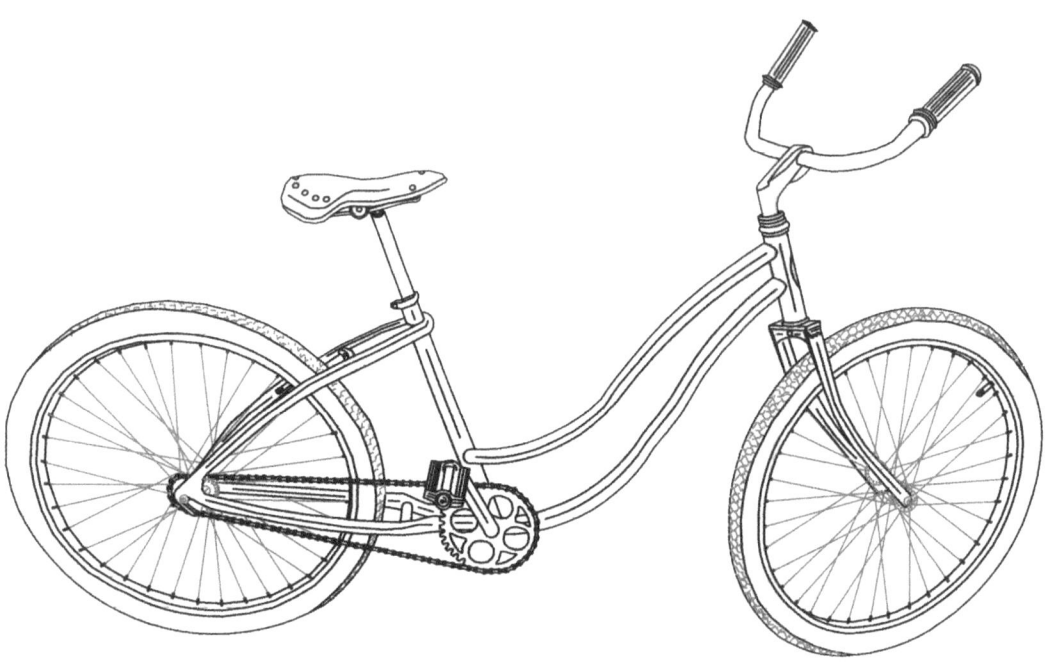

The First Bike

This was the *first* bike: the one that opened the door for me to love and pursue bicycling as a lifelong activity. It ushered me unceremoniously into the realms of the *vélo*, the wheel, the noble bicycle, which would emerge in all its aspects and remain among the great passions in my life. Of course, riding this bike also gave me important opportunities to have experiences of emancipation, feelings of freedom and potential. Even as a kid I gravitated to these. It wasn't just about developing confidence or gaining strength and fitness.

Riding this bike gave me a kid's glimpse of a magical feeling that, as an adult, I describe as bicycling's '*state of bliss*'. It's a point reached during a ride when you're feeling fit and riding strong, relaxed, aware, alert and ready in the moment. At least four senses are saturated, satisfied and stimulated by the physical exertion and visual, auditory and olfactory feasts presented for one's cycling pleasure.[2]

I first caught a kid's glimpse of this experience back then in 1963 and as a lifelong cyclist have had the pleasure of getting a full dose of it many times since. I recognize these moments as

---

2. Of course, this *bicycle bliss* experience ideally includes *no* mechanical mishaps.

some of the best parts of my cycling life and appreciate having the good fortune to be able to write about cycling adventures during which I experienced the serenity of this cycling bliss state as well as those that included thrills and spills, flat tires and everything else.

Growing up in a family with four siblings it was easy to focus first on the independence and the simple rewards that two wheeled freedom from the family scene provided. I had so much *fun* just getting away from home on this *first* bike – with or without friends. Looking back, I can see that I was creating space and the kind of separation that allows a greater measure of independence in defining one's individuality and place within a family. With this bike I could satisfy my *own* curiosity and have my own adventures.

My sister and brothers and I had great times running around *together* during our childhoods. Nevertheless, I can easily recall the sense of autonomy and escape that came with riding Whitey. Coasting down to the park – the wind flowing past my face. Exploring the opposite end of town – on my own. I can see the image of my baseball glove swinging on the handlebars as I climbed the hill to our house after a game. I *loved* this first bike and never crashed or had more than a flat tire while riding it. This bike gave me wings!

Remember son... it's the surprises that 'getcha'

– Dad
  Proprietor of *Dad's Bike Shop* in Albany, California

The Film of Sand (1964)

By mid 1964 I'd grown to nearly five feet tall. Whitey[3] was becoming far too small for me and difficult to ride. I had unceremoniously begun to leave the bike at home, opting to walk to local destinations again. The town center in Pinole, California was nearby and my brothers and I would often make peanut butter sandwiches and walk to the park with our bats, balls, and gloves to meet other kids and play baseball for several hours – calling it quits when dinner time approached.

One Sunday my brother Peter and I were winding our way home after a ballgame when we passed a house where a garage sale was underway. A dull black *Raleigh* 3-speed bicycle stood tall at the back of the two car driveway. Glass dishware and standard 'flea market' items were arrayed on mats spread out over the concrete. The white, paper price tag tied to the bike's handlebars flapped in the wind as if it was waving at me. I could read it from the sidewalk – *$20*. It was a classic *Raleigh 'English Racer'* with steel rimmed, twenty six inch wheels, caliper brakes, fenders and the famous *Sturmey-Archer* rear hub with three internal gears. It even had a speedometer and a generator driven headlight. The shiny chrome reflected a beam of fading sunlight directly into my eyes.

"*Twenty* dollars?" I said to myself, *"that's paper route money."*

"Hey Pete, you know that *route* money you owe me?" It was my older brother's newspaper delivery route but he had always paid me for helping him.

"It's only ten bucks, dummy," he said, "that bike is twenty." He had already seen me looking at it across the driveway.

"Come on, man, you know I'm gonna' pay you back. I'll give it to you by next month."

I knew that between helping him with the newspapers and doing some neighborhood lawn mowing jobs I'd easily have another ten dollars by then.

Forget it – I don't have it," he said. I knew he did.

---

3. *'Whitey'* was the 20 inch wheeled single speed *Schwinn* that I had 'borrowed' permanently from a neighbor a year earlier.

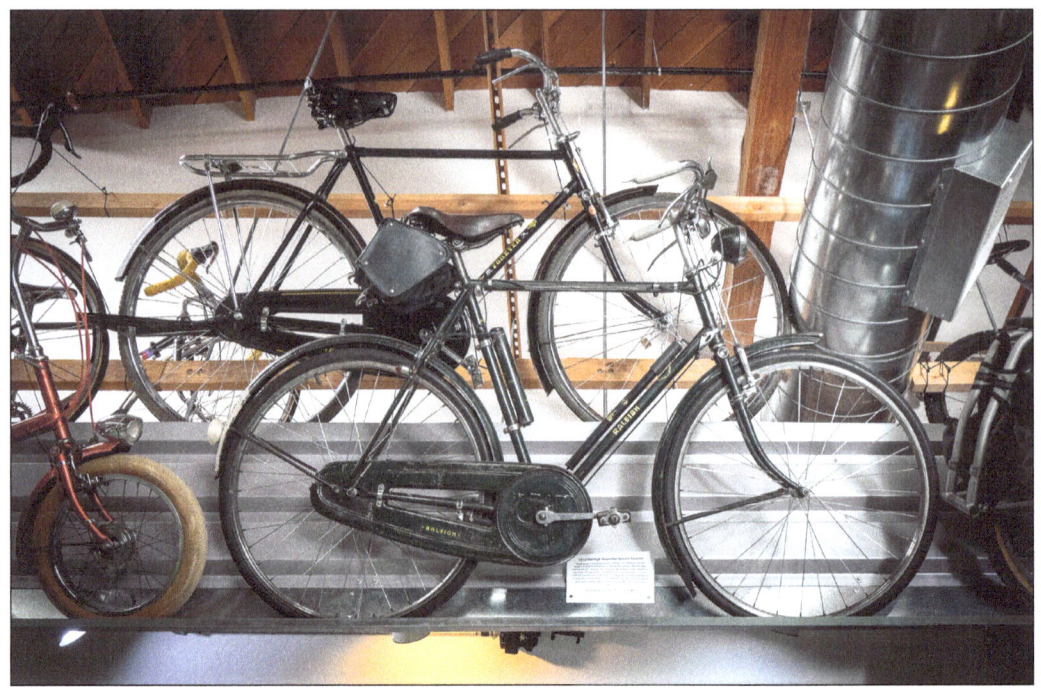

Raleigh 3-speed 'English Racer' – in front of a ***Forever*** 3-speed, its Chinese-made equivalent. *(Courtesy Marin Museum of Bicycling)*

"Come on, Pete, don't mess around; I know you do – ten bucks is nothing to you – come on." I was pleading.

"I said I don't have it, *twerp!*" he repeated.

In the United States, it was kids television's era of *The Three Stooges.* In the mixture of our good clean brotherly fun, my younger brother Tony and I were both used to Pete's impersonations of the *Stooges* leader, Moe Howard, complete with pranks, practical jokes, and name calling, etc. I kept quiet for a few seconds – I didn't want him to get mad.

"You've got it at home," I said. He prided himself on keeping his miniature safe – with a changeable combination lock – full of his paper route money.

Next came the tough love. "Alright, shut up then – I'll give it to you tomorrow." He growled it… like one of *James Cagney's* best gangster lines.

"No, *today*… they might sell it." I was too fast for him. "Hey mister," I quickly asked the man sitting at the card table with the cashbox and a beer, "Are you gonna' be open tomorrow?"

"No, son, we've been out here all weekend and we're closing up at six o'clock," he replied.

"Will you keep that bike for me?" I asked, "I'll be right back."

"Sure thing, but don't forget, I said six o'clock," he replied. I looked at my older brother.

"Pete, let's go – we gotta' hurry up."

"I'm not runnin' three blocks," he said sternly. I started to shuffle sideways towards home.

"Come on, we're gonna' be late for dinner if we don't hurry – I'm runnin'," I said, and took off.

"Stay out of my room! You can't have it until I get there, or I'm gonna' kick your *you-know-what*," he yelled.

He knew I was going to pick the lock on his safe and take the money so I could get the bike and be back in time for dinner. I knew he could reset the combination on the lock and that he would inflict some form of minor punishment for the transgression. I didn't care.

———

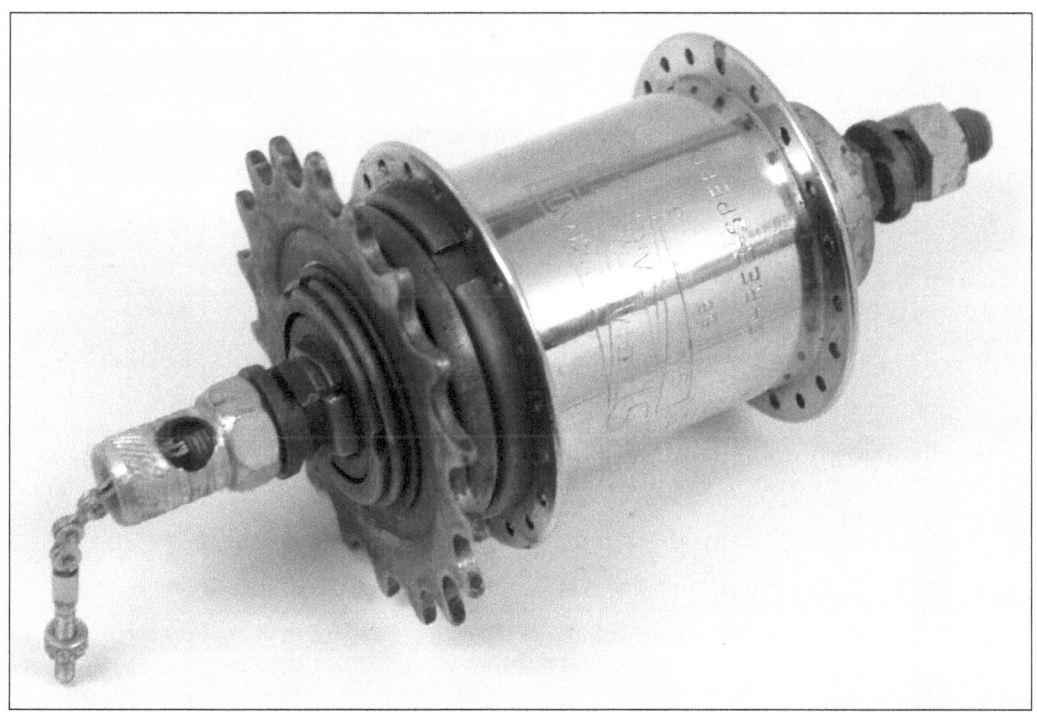

Sturmey-Archer 3-speed hub

Two weekends later I was rolling around Pinole on a bike that fit me! I had cleaned and shined every bit of my 'new' three speed, oiled the chain, pumped up the tires, put a new bulb in the headlight, and continued what eventually became a long tradition of calling my bikes something related to their color. Whitey had passed the torch to '*Blackie*.' I was riding this beauty wherever I went and as often as I could. The 'click – click – clicking' of the *Sturmey-Archer* hub was like music to my ears. I realized and appreciated how quickly a bike ride could put a smile on my face, no matter what my mood. Saturday morning arrived and with my chores and lawn mowing done I was ready to fly once again – this time to visit my school pal Eric in nearby Tara Hills.

In the 1960's Tara Hills was a new, not yet fully built subdivision. There were numerous vacant lots and houses under construction while families were also moving into new tract homes. There were piles of dirt, lumber and construction materials next to cars parked in driveways and along sidewalks. It was here, at the bottom of a steep hill called Marlesta Drive, that the thin layer of loose sand and gravel lay in wait for Blackie and me.

I took off from my house and coasted down to Marlesta Drive. There was a short half block climb up to the crest before Marlesta dropped steeply straight down into Tara Hills so I pedaled hard to gain some momentum as I came up over the top. I flipped the gear shifter into high and began my quarter mile coast down to the bottom where I would make the ninety degree left turn onto Shamrock Drive.

There was no wind but the rush of air past my ears sounded like a small jet roaring down a runway. With no side streets until the bottom of the hill you could really let it out and I picked up a lot of speed quickly. The hub clicks increased their tempo and the wind felt good in my hair. I was easily traveling twenty five miles an hour when I began to brake and prepared to ignore the stop sign as I turned left onto Shamrock. I swung out to the right a bit and followed a fast wide line through the turn, keeping as much speed as possible.

Suddenly, there it was – the almost invisible film of sand was at least twenty feet long and might as well have been oil and water! I realized I was beginning to slide sideways and instinctively tried to remain upright but it was too late to steer away from the parked car directly in my path. I smashed into it sideways at probably fifteen miles an hour, breaking off the side mirror with my right thigh as I catapulted off the bike and over the hood of the car on to the street in front of it. I slid forward along the pavement for a moment and opened my eyes to see my bike bouncing end over end on my left, like a gymnast enthusiastically doing flips. There wasn't a soul around.

I had hit the ground hard enough to scrape my right cheek, both hands and knees, but remained conscious. I'd torn my shirt and pants and the abrasions were already smarting as I picked myself up off the street. Blackie lay ten feet away with the back wheel still spinning. My right leg hurt something fierce as I stepped gingerly toward my seriously damaged bicycle. My knee was on fire. "Damn it," I exclaimed.

The front wheel was now shaped like a teardrop, the steel rim broken. The fork was bent back at the crown, and the frame tubes were badly crimped right behind the stem. I picked it up and twisted the handlebars back to their proper position. The saddle was shredded on the side that had scraped along the pavement.

The front wheel wouldn't roll. Besides the tire being flat the bent wheel could no longer rotate through the fork blades. "Ah, *MAN*!" I yelled to no one. It was becoming crystal clear to me that my *Raleigh* was a wreck. As I began the long steep walk, dragging and carrying the bike back up Marlesta Drive to my house, it was also becoming clear that my right thigh had taken a big impact. I was limping with every step.

I was glad there was no one around. I was hurt but I felt embarrassed. I was bleeding and my 'new' bike was bent and broken. When I finally reached the crest where I'd begun this ill-fated descent I saw one of the neighborhood moms in her yard watering the lawn.

"Are you alright?" she said. It was a stupid question spoken with genuine concern.

"What do you think? Do I *look* alright?" I thought – I was mad that someone had seen me.

"Yes, Mrs. Miller," I responded. "I just took a little spill down at the bottom of Marlesta. I'm okay. My bike's kinda' wrecked though." Feigning a smile so she would think I was okay hurt my cheek. Staring down at the bike, it seemed there was no way I could fix the frame.

"Looks like you scraped yourself up quite a bit," she continued, preferring to focus on me, "Can I help you?"

"No, thank you, Mrs. Miller, I gotta' get home," I said. As I dragged my dead bike around the last corner near our house I began thinking about what might happen when I got there.

I went in through the back yard gate and leaned Blackie against the fence. Quietly slipping into the garage, my plan was to clean up quickly, then change my pants and shirt.

"Ouch!" It was either the fiery abrasions or the dark purple bruise that was already forming on the top of my entire right thigh that drew another groan. I looked in the mirror my dad had near his workbench and saw the red, silver dollar-size abrasion on my cheek.

I knew I wouldn't be able to hide what had happened for long. Just then, the door from the kitchen opened and in walked Pete. He saw my cheek immediately.

"What the heck did you do now – get in a fight? You're in trouble." He was always like this until he knew what was going on.

"Nothin'," I said.

"You're gonna' get it if you don't tell me what happened," he replied. I was scraped and sore, my cheek was stinging and my thigh hurt.

"I crashed my bike." He was silent for a moment – as if forced to feel some compassion.

"Where is it?" he asked, "You look like you totaled it."

"Out by the trash," I answered, "I did."

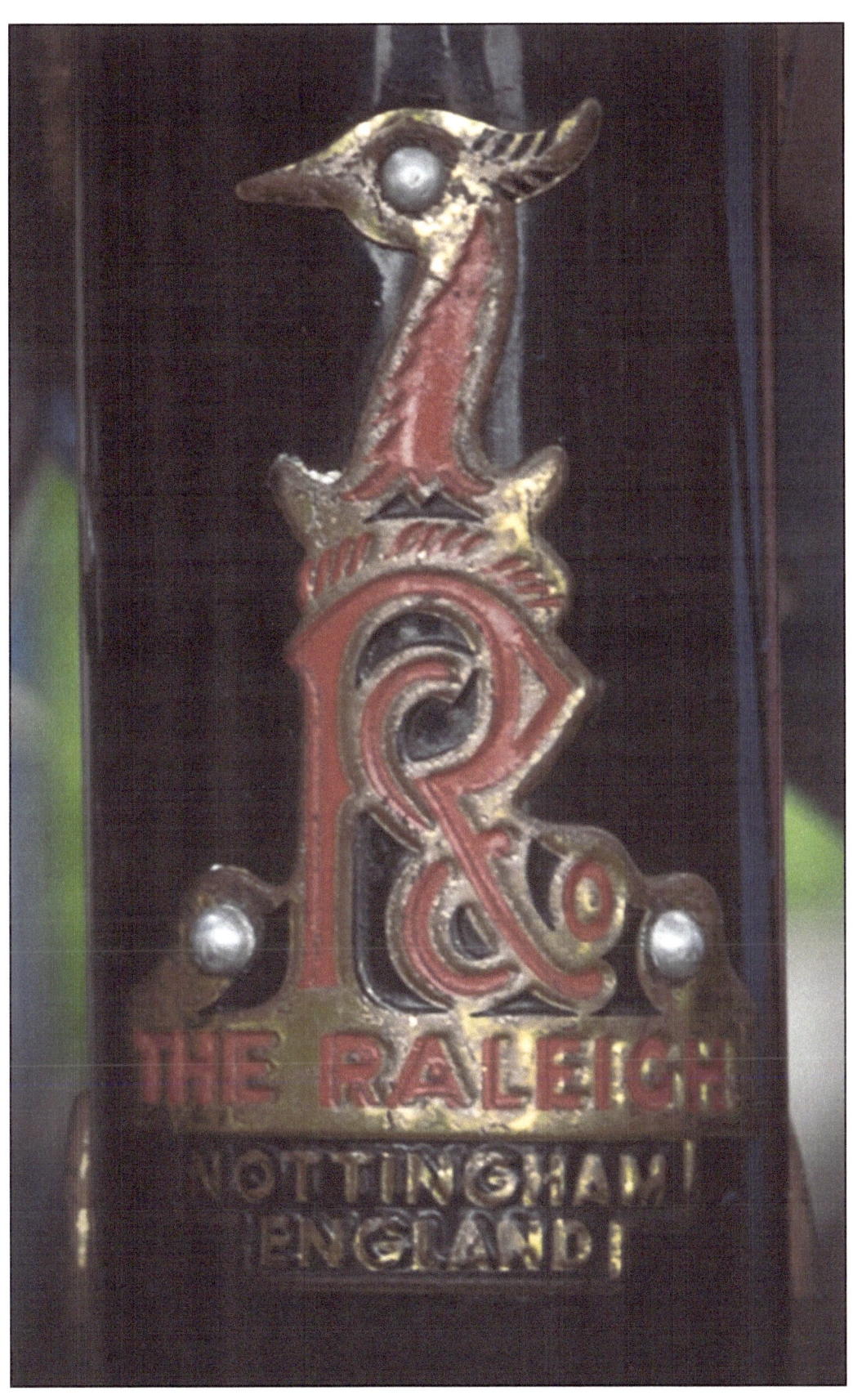

Vintage *Raleigh* frame detail – metal head tube badge (1979)

He went down so fast it was like the rug got pulled out from under him!

– MOE HOWARD
  Actor, film and television star of The Three Stooges

Slip-Sliding Away: Oil on the Mountain (1983)

It was the fall of 1983. October – the month that my brother Pete died at a mere thirty three years of age – a month that saddened the birthdays of my many October-born family members. That same month I had my wisdom teeth removed and my girlfriend began a two month sojourn in southeast Asia. It was a *wrenching* and painful month but I managed to turn the wrenching around. I put together my first real road racing bike. The frameset – a new royal blue *Colnago Superissimo;* the components – *Campagnolo Super Record* throughout with custom built *Velosport* wheels.[4] *Ma Che Bella Bicicletta!*

I had been planning to build a new bike for months and had already purchased the $500 frameset at a deep discount from *Bike Nashbar*, a big shop on Wilshire Boulevard in Santa Monica, California. *Colnago* – I had always wanted an Italian racing bike and in my world, this was the frame of a stallion. It was easy to convince myself that it deserved 'top shelf' components and a custom wheelset. After riding years and hundreds of miles on my trusty $150 *Puegeot* I knew I would greatly appreciate a more expensive bike. I purchased everything I needed and used my time off during 'wisdom tooth' week to assemble my new steel and aluminum thoroughbred. It had cost a pretty penny – about *$900* by the time I was rolling – but I didn't care. I now had the fastest, best looking bike I'd ever owned.

I was living in Sausalito in 1983, where riding along the flatlands adjacent to San Francisco Bay on my new *Colnago*, 'Super Blue,' meant riding *fast*. It was partly because of the racing gears I was pedaling. The *Campagnolo Super Record* crankset on my new bike had a 44 tooth inner chainring, making the lowest gear not so low. The local steep terrain around southern Marin County instantly became quite challenging. Still being naïve about racing

---

4. *Velosport* was the venerable 'pro' bike shop operated by local legend Peter Rich in Berkeley, California.

gear ratios, I hadn't yet realized that a 39 tooth inner chainring is often considered an appropriate gear for climbing steep terrain. Even professional cyclists at that time were more likely to use a 40 or 42 tooth inner chainring for most racing.

Nevertheless, having gotten a discount on the *Campagnolo* components, I resolved to just 'get used' to the gearing that I had. Soon I realized that if I remained seated and pulled back on the handlebars, I could make it up any of the steeper hills I was used to riding at the time, including Mt. Tamalpais.[5] I became a decent climber and began to crave those weekend mornings when I would head up and over Panoramic Highway to Stinson Beach and north to Point Reyes Station or south to Muir Beach.

This particular Saturday was one of those spectacular 'Indian Summer,' October days. It was warm and breezy. Songbirds made their morning calls and the smells of sage, chemise and manzanita were in the wind – thick and enveloping – like aromas in an old wine cellar. I climbed silently up the Panoramic Highway, thinking about my brother and my girlfriend… and how wonderfully tight and responsive the steering on my new bike was. Despite all the effort I was smiling as I reached the 1,500 foot crest at Pantoll Station and began my descent toward Stinson Beach.

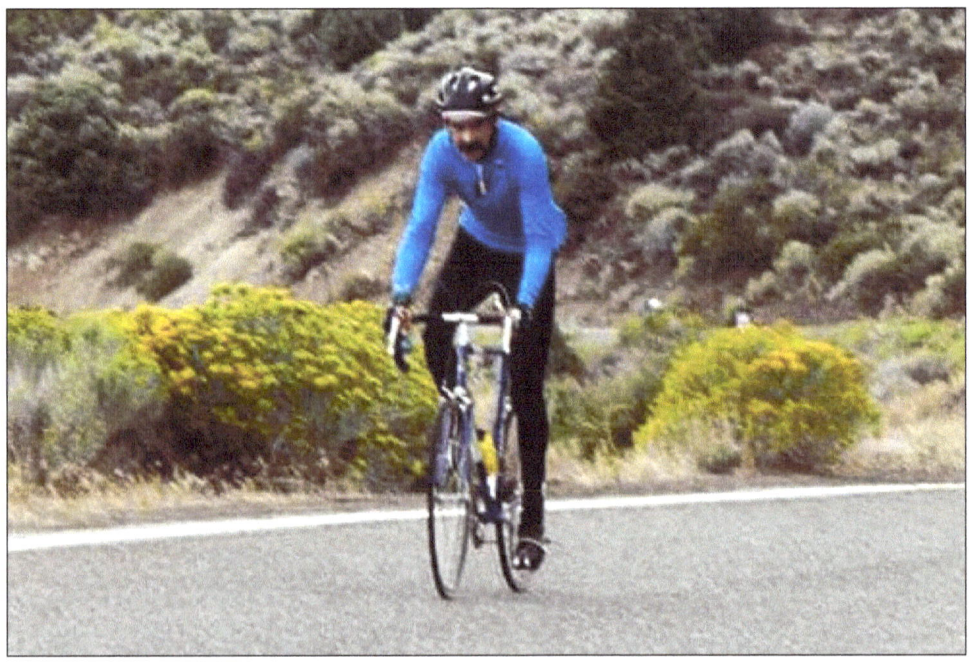

Climbing on 'Super Blue' – aka my 1983 *Colnago Superissimo*

---

5. The parking lot at East Peak on Mount Tamalpais is reached after a final 18% incline.

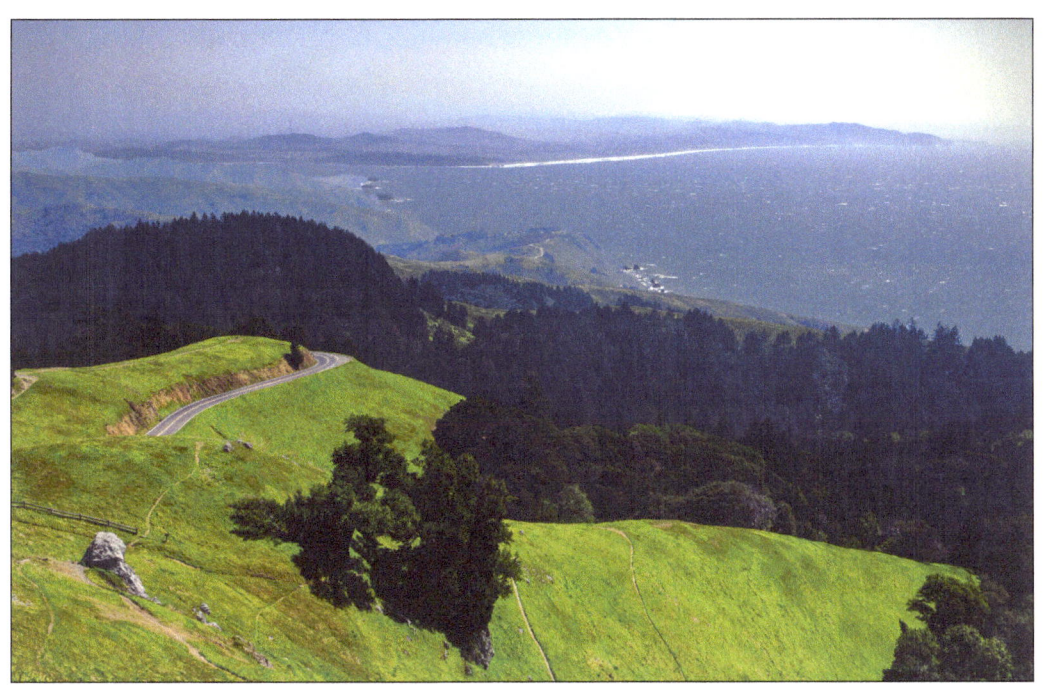

View towards San Francisco from Mount Tamalpais, Marin County

Most serious cyclists would likely describe the descent to the coast on Panoramic Highway as somewhat technical – especially if they enjoy a fast downhill run as 'payback' for their effort on the uphill sections. Sweeping sunlit curves are interspersed with tight, shady, hairpin turns at the creek crossings. Riders learn to see the best line of pavement to follow as they speed down the hill, rolling with maximum momentum. The 'best' line changes, of course, depending on the road conditions or even traffic but once cyclists become familiar with the terrain they can relax a bit and 'let it out' on the downhill sections – knowing when to 'freewheel' and when to 'feather' the brakes. But you don't usually expect fresh motor oil on the downhill switchback turns! At least I didn't… before then.

The Panoramic Highway emerges from the dense oak woodland on a wide promontory about a mile or so above Stinson Beach. The serpentine bedrock is exposed in the steep road cuts forming a double set of tight, switchback turns that bring the road down to the town at about sea level. The sun was reflecting off the shiny green surfaces directly into my eyes. I blinked and shook my head to get some of the sweat out of my eyes and saw two female riders single file up ahead, speeding their way down to the coast.

"Good descenders," I thought to myself. I was a hundred feet or so behind them and made no effort to close the gap. I could see they were wearing the matched jerseys of a team or cycling club. These girls were serious riders and sped down the hill, easily staying ahead of me. The number of strong women riders was increasing and I admired any racers and endurance riders. I figured I might see them in town where I could say hello and see what they were up to. They began to slow as they approached the first set of hairpin curves. I was gaining ground on them as they rounded the tight turn and disappeared from view.

"I guess I'll just catch up," I thought. Both women were only fifty feet ahead of me when they came back into view. I prepared to lean into the lower pair of tight switchbacks as they both dropped out of site again. Coming out of the turn I was suddenly shocked to see that both of them had somehow crashed! They were still lying on the ground just ahead of me, struggling to get up and untangle their bikes. Instinctively, I began to sit up but in an instant, both my front and rear wheels slid sideways as if someone had 'pulled the rug out from under me.' I immediately slammed to the ground on my left side and began sliding down the road head first on my back. It was still the era of toe clips and straps and somehow I managed to lift the bike with my legs and feet until I stopped sliding.

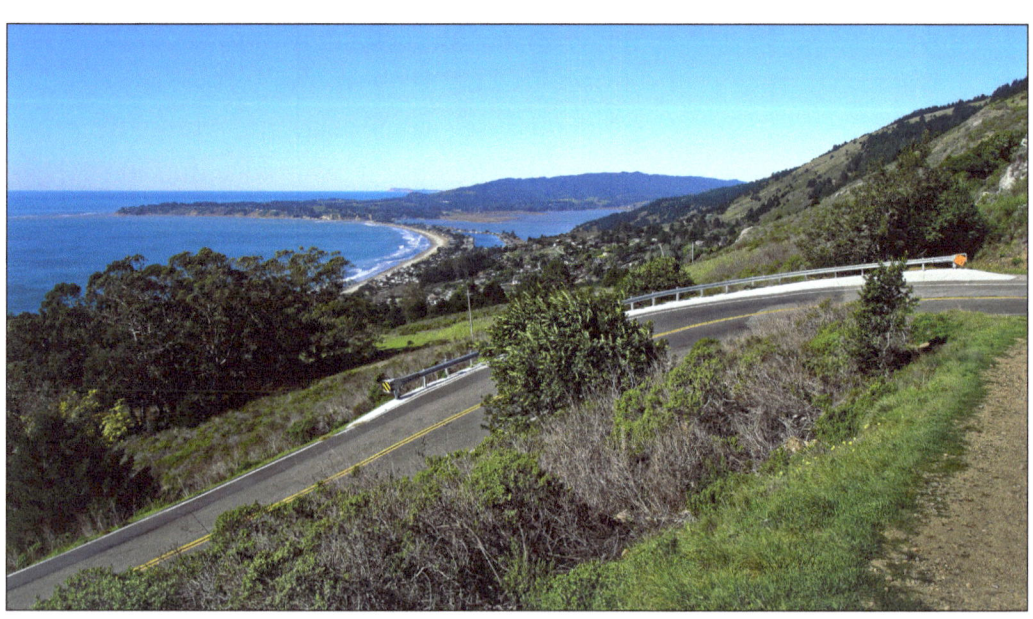

Switchback turn on the Panoramic Highway above Stinson Beach and the Bolinas Mesa

My first thought was "Good thing there are no cars coming right now." I got myself and the bike over to the side of the road as quickly as possible.

"Are you okay?" one of the girls called out to me.

"I think so," I said, tentatively. I was trying to figure out what had happened. Nothing felt broken but I had torn my jersey and shorts in the slide. "How about you guys?" I asked.

"Just scrapes and bruises," the brunette one who turned out to be Jennifer replied, "Your jersey is ripped – what *was* that up there?"

I looked my bike over as I rolled it down slowly to where they were standing. I smelled motor oil on my torn jersey and it looked like there was oil on both of my tires. I touched it and put my finger to my nose.

"Somebody's car must have been leaking," I said, "There's oil on the switchback. Are you guys too hurt to ride?" I asked, "Are your bikes okay?" I had distinguished them by hair color initially and the brunette who turned out to be Jennifer said "no" while her lighter haired friend who turned out to be Kathy simultaneously said "yes." We all chuckled for a moment – I knew Jennifer had answered the first question and Kathy, the second.

"You scraped the back of your shoulder." The brunette who turned out to Jennifer had noticed, "Do you want me to look at it before we ride down?"

I was getting a windbreaker out of my pack so I could cover the silver dollar-size abrasion which was already beginning to sting. I felt a bruise forming on the inside of my right thigh where it had hit the frame's top tube. Amazingly, my bike was unscathed except for scrapes on the tire sidewalls and the outside of the left pedal. I looked her right in the eyes.

"That's cool, I'm alright – it's not really bleeding. I'll just cover it with my jacket and wash it when I get home," I replied. For some typical – but illogical – reason I had always felt vulnerable right after a mishap like this. I didn't want her to think that I was hurt and opted to change the subject. "What's your name, anyway?"

"Jennifer," she replied, and quickly introduced her companion. "This is my friend, Kathy." They both looked very fit.

"Sorry it was these conditions but nice to meet you, Jennifer. Hi Kathy – I'm Jonathan."

Get on your bikes and ride!

– Freddie Mercury
  Legendary singer, musician, composer and front man for the rock band *Queen*

Those First Scratches! (1983)

It was late December of 1983. I'd been riding my prized new *Colnago Superissimo* for two months – getting used to the bike's racing gears. The lowest gears were not so low but what a beautiful blue color! There wasn't a smudge anywhere. I still hadn't figured out that a 44/53 tooth crankset just isn't that well suited for the steep climbs of the San Francisco Bay Area but I was riding a ton and adjusting well. I was fit and enthusiastic. The bike I called *'Super Blue'* was performing like a true thoroughbred!

Christmas was approaching and besides immersing myself in year end work projects, I was spending a lot of my late afternoons riding along the bay shoreline in southern Marin County and doing longer solo rides each weekend. Living on a houseboat in Sausalito at that time had many advantages and one of them was the convenient access to so many great cycling routes – there was something for whatever type of riding I preferred.

But none of them are preferred when you're hungover... and that's what I was this particular Saturday morning. Friday night drinks with work colleagues to celebrate the season had involved more drinks than I'm used to – without much food – at one of their Sausalito apartments – followed by a half hour in a hot tub sipping prosecco! Needless to say I wasn't in the best form to do a training ride that next morning but managed to suit up about ten o'clock, intending to ride a thirty mile loop from Sausalito to Stinson Beach and back – via Muir Beach. I had the naïve expectation that I would 'sweat it out' over a couple of hours.

I've probably been *really* 'hungover' just a handful of times in my life – this happened to be one of them. Not being a big drinker has its benefits in that you don't go through this hangover 'stuff' often. On the other hand, if I had known better I doubt I would have headed up over the 1,500 foot shoulder of Mount Tamalpais that foggy, wet morning. Luckily, I was wearing all my cold weather clothing because I began to sweat profusely as soon as I started the climb. I was glad I knew the least strenuous route up the mountain through Mill Valley. I could tell right away this was going to be a long thirty miles.

Those who know the profile of Mount Tamalpais are familiar with the 'stair step' character of the terrain on the Panoramic Highway, where a rider climbs steeply at times and more gradually – along topographic contours – at others. The average four percent gradient from Sausalito to Pantoll Station combines lots of seven or eight percent segments with several short, steeper inclines *and* some nearly level sections along the ridgelines above Muir Woods National Monument and within Mount Tamalpais State Park. Overall, it's a 'tough' ride – but not *that* tough – the flat spots provide some respite along the way.

Well, that's how it usually works… this particular morning it felt like a '*grind*' – all work. I was anticipating each one of those flatter sections and every one of them felt as slow as the climbs did. The steep pitches had me out of the saddle immediately! I was spending a lot of time in my low gears and finally got some relief when I emerged from the fog at Bootjack Camp. I felt the rush of warm morning sunlight and unzipped my jacket. My jersey was soaked. I rode on and stopped at Pantoll Station where I refilled my water bottle and drank some of the applesauce, brown sugar and water mixture that I carried in my second bottle. The banana that I brought along would wait. I took off my jacket and hung it across my handlebars while I sat in the sun thinking about the rest of the ride.

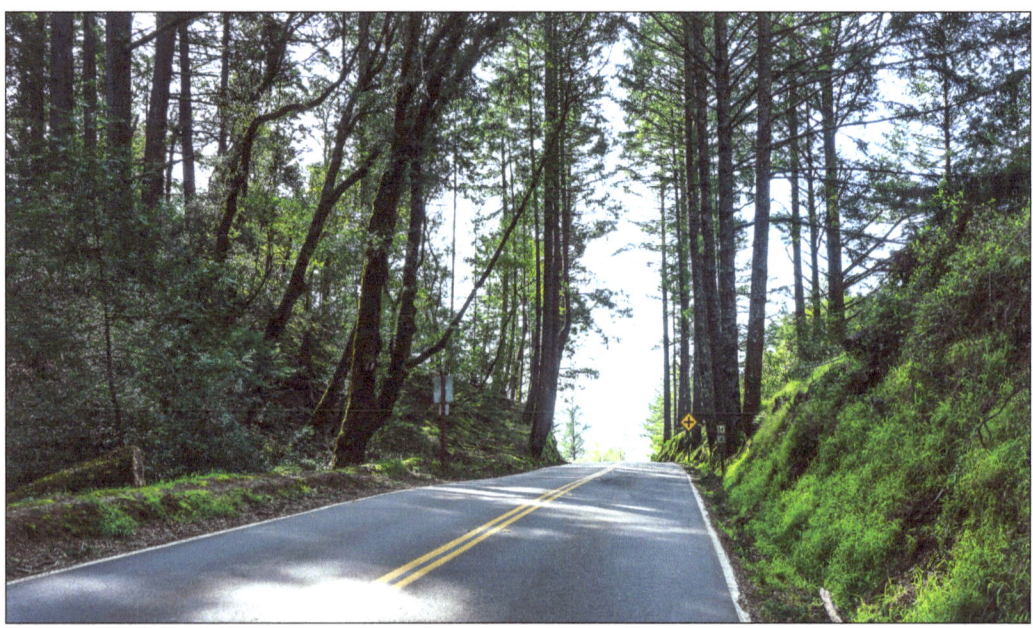

Approaching Pantoll Station along the Panoramic Highway, Marin County

The Panoramic Highway descends steeply from Pantoll Station to Highway 1 on the coast, just south of Stinson Beach. On a clear day the shade of the switchbacks through the redwoods finally gives way to sweeping views of the Pacific Ocean and the Bolinas Lagoon. However, at least for now, this was no clear day at the coast. Even as I sat basking in the sun at an elevation of 1,500 feet, wisps of fog were drifting in below from the west, making their way inland and up the ravines into the redwoods. I put my jacket on and got ready for a slow and steady downhill run to the coast.

As I pedaled out of the parking lot I saw the Park Ranger sitting in the sun on the steps of the Visitor Center reading a newspaper. A few folded pages of advertisements flapped gently in the breeze where he held them under one of his boot heels. My sun warmed hungover brain realized that I needed that newspaper – not to read but to put under my shirt – an old motorcyclist's trick for keeping the upper body warm. I greeted the ranger and asked if I could take some of his paper's advertisements.

"Sure," he said, handing me a couple of sections. He looked like he knew what I was doing as I slid the paper under the front of my jersey and rode away.

The slow, cold roll down the hill to Stinson Beach was just *that*. There was no traffic and the pavement was fairly dry. I freewheeled into the foggy mist and feathered my front brake as I contemplated the fact that I had just committed to riding *20 more miles!* It meant climbing another 1000 feet in order to get to Muir Beach, then over the hill to Tamalpais Valley Junction and home to Sausalito. I reached Stinson Beach and decided to head to the beach cafe for a coffee before starting my journey back.

The coastal fog in California often lifts slightly as the morning sun rises. It may not burn off entirely until early afternoon but depending on where you are, the view of the ocean and visibility at the beach elevation can remain several miles beneath the fog bank. Stinson Beach is one of those great spots where the natural topography and sun can also interact in a way that creates occasional breaks in the fog near the center of town and the State Beach. This was one of those days and the Saturday morning chill was already abating at the beach. The cafe was open. I perched myself on a warm spot where I glimpsed patches of blue sky increasing above and proceeded to enjoy my cappuccino.

Off came the jacket *and* jersey, which I hung in the sun on the chair next to me. Some of the newspaper pages were already wet after being pressed inside my clothing and I tossed the ones that were soaked with sweat. The cafe clock showed almost 11 am. My hangover was abating but I was super thirsty. I decided to look over some of the ads while I gradually ate my banana and finished my coffee. The sun felt good and I settled in for some additional 'reptilian' moments before the climb south to Muir Beach.

Hot drink, warm sunny spot, reading uninteresting stuff – it was a recipe for dozing and the next thing I knew I was awakened by newspaper pages flapping in my face. It had been a mere fifteen minutes but my inadvertent 'catnap' was over. My half finished drink was on its side and coffee had dripped down the table legs. I snapped out of my momentary snooze, used the newspaper to wipe up what remained of the spill and put on my salt streaked, sun-dried jersey. It was time to go.

I filled my water bottle and began pedaling back to the highway. The ride back from Stinson Beach would be a steady, steep, 500 foot ascent of the coastal bluff followed by a likewise steep but very fast descent to Muir Beach and then one last climb of about 600 foot, winding steadily past the San Francisco Zen Center's Green Gulch farm.

As I headed south it was quickly back to 'grinding' on the steeply inclined section of road cut directly into the coastal bluff. The fog was lifting. I passed Steep Ravine Campground and glimpsed the western San Francisco skyline in the distance. Point San Pedro was visible at the horizon. It had warmed up a bit and my dripping sweat resembled a leaking faucet. Climbing past the Steep Ravine trailheads I finally reached a flat section where Highway 1 turns inland before crossing Lone Tree Creek.

In Marin County, California's coastal Highway 1 is different than in areas such as Mendocino or Big Sur. There are fewer bridges over the narrow ravines and streams that drain directly to the ocean. Instead, the highway alignment typically turns inland following the terrain and descends to cross a stream culvert before climbing back towards the coast and continuing along the bluff. Even when traffic is light and the road surface is

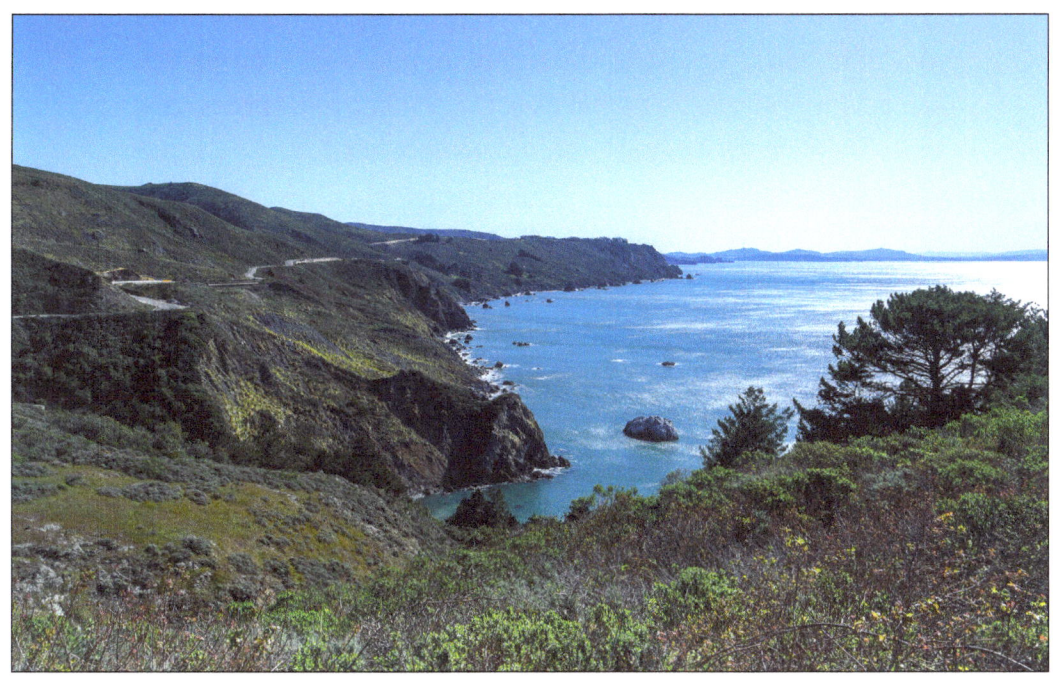

View towards Hwy 1 and San Francisco (on horizon) from south of Stinson Beach, Marin County

smooth a seasoned cyclist must still pay close attention, checking their speed on the descent inland and making sure to select the proper low gear *before* the switchback turn that begins the climb west to the next section of road along the coastal headland. There's an art and a science to maintaining one's momentum through these tight turns and abrupt slope changes.

It's good thing I was riding alone that day. In my hazy state I wasn't much of a role model for cyclists learning to negotiate sharp turns with abrupt gains in elevation. Instead, I proceeded to embarrass myself in solitude *and* put the *first* scratches on my new bike! I was so relieved to be rolling downhill I automatically shifted gears to my big chainring without really thinking about what was ahead. As I slowed to cross the short, level, culverted switchback turn over Lone Creek I realized my mistake.

It was too late – three things happened all at once. The grade steepened, my cadence dropped abruptly and when I stood on the pedals – trying to keep my momentum – my rear wheel immediately lost traction on the wet pavement. I attempted to shift to a lower gear but all I could manage was a single, *attempted* pedal revolution – grinding the chain on the front derailleur. I quickly came to a complete stop, panting from trying everything just to keep pushing further to a spot where I could double back and shift into my lowest gear.

It must have looked like a failed 'track stand' when I tipped over sideways, landing on my left forearm and hip. It seemed to happen in slow motion. Luckily, my cleated shoes had come out of the 'toe clips and straps' still commonly used at the time. I got myself off the ground and the first thing I thought was "*Man*, I'm glad nobody saw that!" I was unhurt by the slow speed fall but still winded from the extreme effort.

I caught my breath and rolled my bike to the shoulder of the road so I could look it over and shift the gears back to the inner chain ring. Embarrassment was becoming anger. Not only did I now have grease on my hands but I saw that my water bottle had popped out and rolled off the road. As I put my bike against a tree I saw that the leather at the back of the saddle was scratched and torn at the corner.

"Damn it!" I said out loud to no one. I was pissed at myself for getting the first scratches on my new *Colnago* while tipping over as if I was part of a bicycle comedy act. It was entirely avoidable. Everything could have been different – my approach to the turn, my focus and of course, what had gone on the night before. I retrieved my water bottle and returned to my bike, noticing the handlebars had twisted slightly when I fell. As I rotated them back I saw that the left brake lever was also scratched. "God*damn* it!" My anger erupted again.

The 'upside' was that my hangover was now completely gone. The adrenaline, the sweat… and maybe the realization that true mistakes cannot be *undone* — only learned from – operated to my benefit for the rest of the ride. I can't say I enjoyed it but I used the energy of the moment and rode on with steady resolve and maybe a bit more than my usual amount of caution on the tight hairpin turns and rapid descent into Muir Beach. I could feel the scratches on my brake lever every time I slowed down. It was early afternoon but I'd had enough for the day. My frustration and fatigue settled in.

I made the hard right turn at the base of the hill and passed the Pelican Inn before beginning the last sustained climb of the day, winding steadily on Highway 1 to its intersection with Panoramic Highway. I was mentally and physically done with the day's effort as I reached the crest and began my last descent to Tamalpais Valley Junction. Breezes off the bay became light headwinds as I cruised along the bike path to Sausalito.

Once home I couldn't help but reflect heavily on the day. The scratches were cosmetic and looked less important to me, even as I cleaned up the bike and washed the grease off my hands. But that wasn't the point. It wasn't so much about the bike. Standing in the shower later on I found myself repeating the words: *Do stupid things – stupid things happen.*

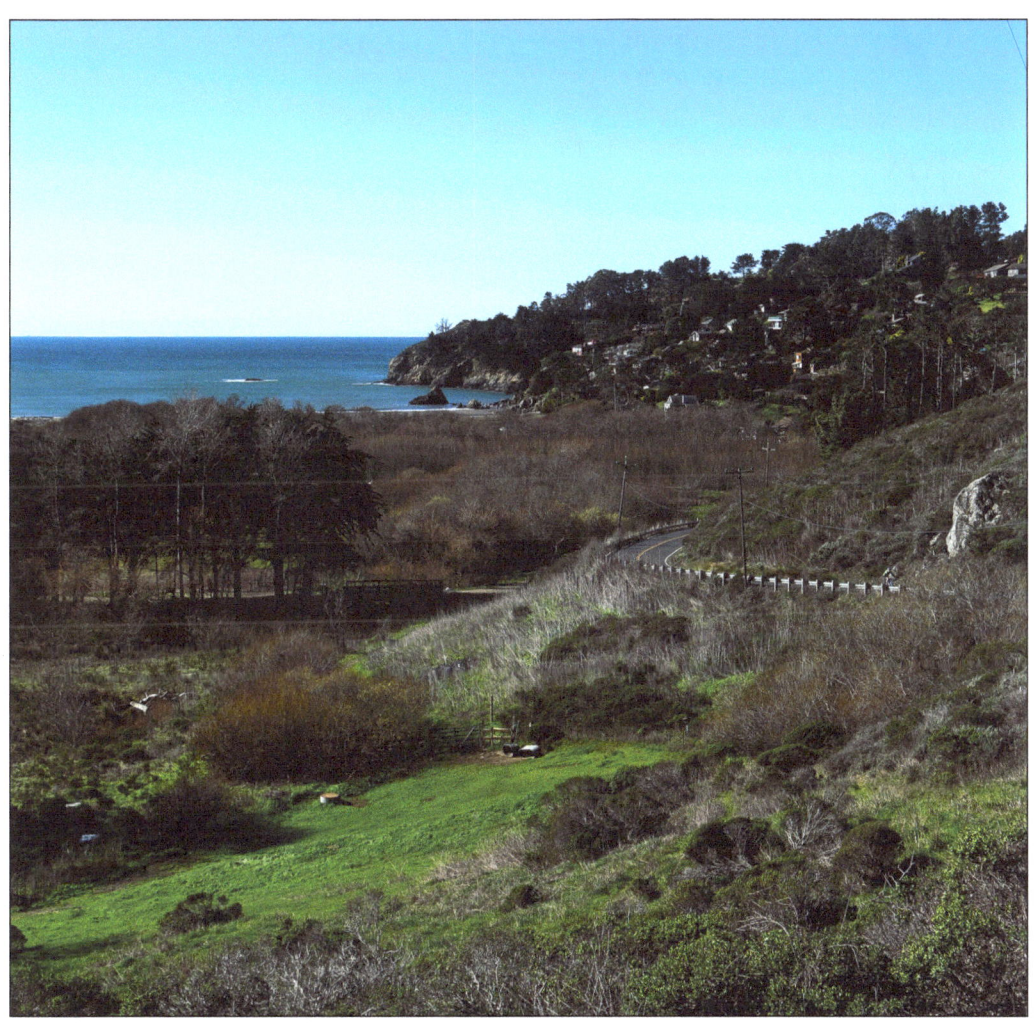

View towards Muir Beach and Hwy 1, Marin County

Don't look for a turn signal or the driver's glance – keep an eye on the car's right front wheel

– TONY TOM
  Longtime proprietor of *A Bicycle Odyssey* in Sausalito, California

Truckin' through Sausalito (1984)

It was something I would never consider doing today. Now in 2025, I'm wondering 'What the hell were you thinking?' Nevertheless, it was the late spring of 1984 – I was twenty nine years old, still defiant and young – and very fit. I was feeling strong and preparing to ride from San Francisco to see the Olympic Games in Los Angeles one month later! There I was – riding my *Colnago* racing bike invincibly along Bridgeway through Sausalito towards the houseboat where I lived at Waldo Pt. Harbor.

Tourist traffic was thicker than usual due to the hot weather and the art festival was taking place along the bay. Rolling along the flats in the bike lane I was steadily passing cars – all forced to inch along, stuck in a single idling column of 'stop and go' movement. The smell of exhaust from an old truck up ahead had permeated the already stagnant shoreline air. I wasn't happy about being forced to breathe the smoke.

I passed a Sausalito Police Car, cruising along in the flow of traffic. The windows were down and the officer riding 'shotgun' gave me a wave.

"Ride safe," he called out as I passed the patrol car.

"I already am," I thought. Not only was I just ambling along at less than ten miles an hour, I'd also gotten a helmet, which I'd started wearing on my longer training rides. I had it on.

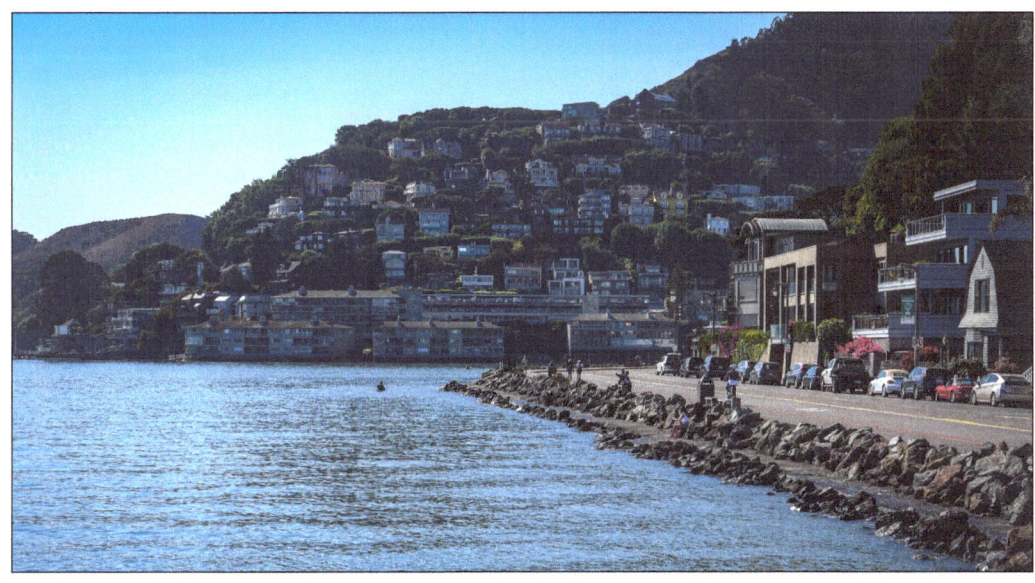

View towards Bridgeway along Sausalito's waterfront

A few moments later, I was coming up alongside the rear of the smoking truck. My instinct was to accelerate past the truck as quickly as possible in order to get away from the noxious exhaust fumes. However, destiny prevailed and before I had time to increase my pace I was suddenly living through one of any cyclist's worst nightmares. The pickup driver didn't look, didn't signal, didn't *see* me and began to turn right – cutting me off! I was pinched to the curb and forced to turn quickly right in order to avoid a collision. Fortunately, I had enough room to make the turn on to the cross street.

"Hey! HEY! HEYYY! What are you *doing*?" I was yelling at the driver as loud as I could, while I made the abrupt turn alongside of the truck. I came to a stop and the truck did, too. His passenger-side window was down.

"Man, where'd you learn how to drive? Use your turn signals!" I was feeling adrenaline.

"Yeah? Ride your bike on the sidewalk *like you're supposed to*?" He yelled back.

"I've got just as much right to the street as you do… you ever heard of the Vehicle Code?" I had said my peace and noticed the rifle rack in the rear truck window. It was a case of some 'redneck' attitude… right there in the notoriously liberal southern Marin County!

"What are you – *a cop*?" He snickered, leaning forward to see me more directly through the passenger window.

"Don't think so, but I sure am." A deep voice came from behind on my left. "And my partner here – he's a cop, too." The redneck's snicker disappeared.

The patrol car had turned right and stopped behind us unnoticed. Both Sausalito Police officers were walking towards us. The one who had been driving went straight towards the driver's door. "Good afternoon sir, can I see your license and registration, please?" The other officer was headed towards me.

"Are you okay?" he asked me. It was the same officer who had called out "Ride safe."

"Yeah, I stayed upright. I guess I'm still pissed that it happened," I said.

"Don't worry about that... Do you live around here?" He inquired. "Can I take a quick look at your driver's license, please?"

"Over on Gate 5 Road," I replied, grabbing my wallet from my back jersey pocket. I handed him my license and he glanced at it quickly before giving it right back to me.

"Mr. Van Coops, I just want to ask you again if you're physically okay – I mean, uninjured."

"Yeah, I'm fine," I said.

"What about your bike?" He continued, "Everything okay with the bike?"

"My bike is fine too," I said, "I managed to avoid tipping over."

"Okay then, if you're not injured, and your bike's okay, there's no reason for you to stay. My partner and I will take care of the incident report for this guy's smoking vehicle and moving violations since we witnessed both, so you're good to go ahead and roll."

"Okay," I said. No question about it – he was a real 'take charge' kind of police officer.

As I rode home I couldn't help reflect on his call to "ride safe," and how fortunate I was not to have been going faster when the truck suddenly turned in front of me. Though I wasn't sure what could have resulted from a collision like that at speed – as destiny would have it – I was to find out while racing in a triathlon at Lake Tahoe the following year. There, another young truck driver would suddenly turn right, directly through the race course in front of me, causing a serious collision and major, life changing injuries.

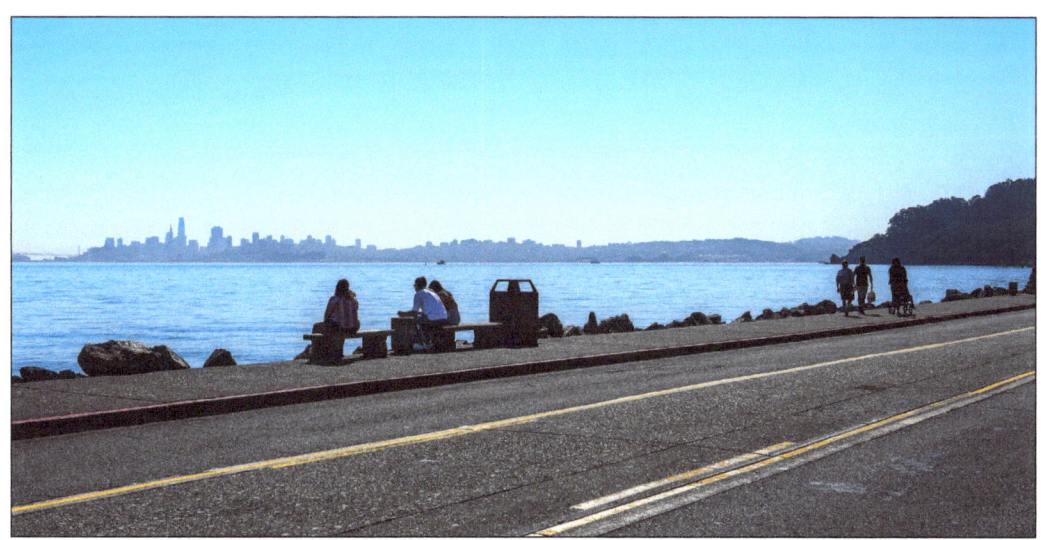

View towards San Francisco from Bridgeway on Sausalito's waterfront

I ride a lot [6]

– Eddy Merckx
Belgian professional cycling hero and five time winner of the *Tour de France*

---

6. Eddy Merckx's response to being asked how he trained.

Cycling to Los Angeles for the Summer Olympic Games (1984)

1984 was a great cycling year for me, one of the best of *many* in a life of cycling now spanning sixty years. I'd assembled my first real racing bike, a *Colnago Superissimo*, during the fall of 1983 and had been training intensively all winter and into the spring of the New Year on my beautiful royal blue thoroughbred. My *Superissimo* was superb!

1984 was also the year that the summer games of the XXIII Olympiad were held in Los Angeles and I became determined to carry out an ambitious plan. Not only would I attend the track cycling events and watching the men's and women's road races, but I would *ride my bike* as a means of getting to Los Angeles! The logistics for such a trip were complicated but I had a three week vacation planned and enough friends and family willing to help me. I was convinced that the numerous details would get handled.

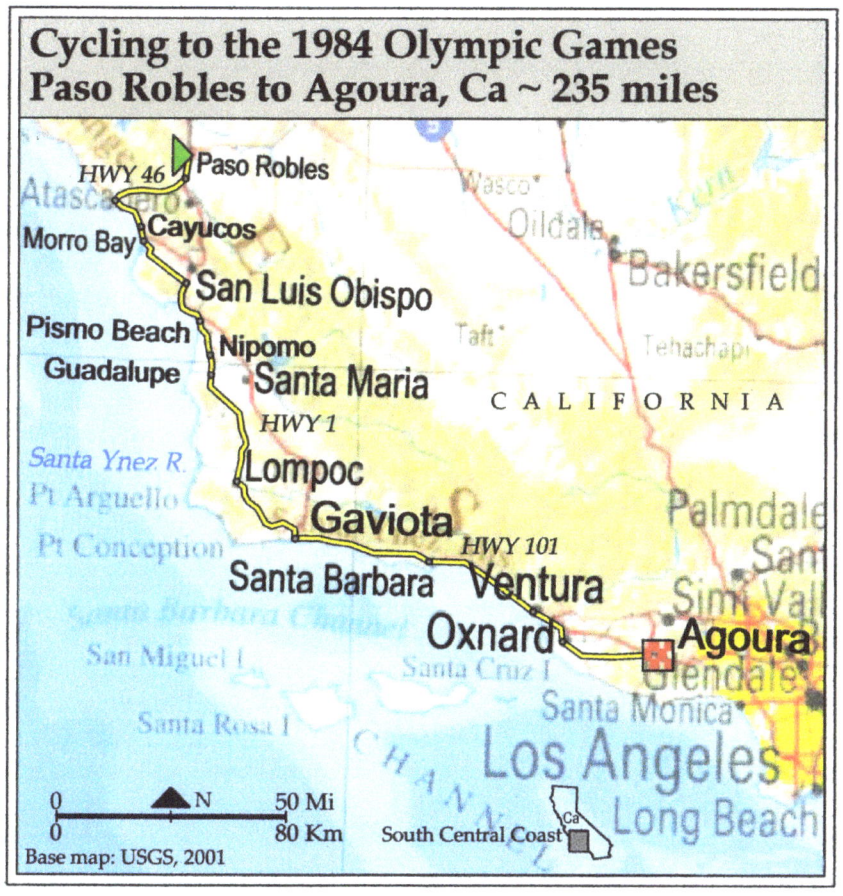

They did... the planning gradually became a consuming effort, developing to a crescendo of activities as the year progressed. Summer arrived and my momentum began to shift from preparation to action. By the fourteenth of July, I had done everything I could – I was ready and fit for the trip. It was to be one of my best ever cycling adventures – beginning with a memorable week of riding about 250 miles along California's central coast.

The Olympic cycling events were to be held in late July and early August, making it perfect to leave San Francisco in mid July and arrive at my sister's house in southern California a few days before attending the Opening Ceremonies. My basic plan was to ride a series of segments down the coast punctuated by overnight accommodations with family or friends. The daily distances would vary – most being within a range of 30 to 80 miles.

July 19th: Paso Robles to Cayucos (28 mi.)

My ride began in earnest in Paso Robles, northern San Luis Obispo County. I began rolling west along Highway 46 towards my brother's place located on the coast, north of the seaside town of Cayucos. No doubt I looked a bit strange – like a 'top-heavy' bike tourist carrying a rucksack stuffed with gear, while riding an Italian racing bike. There were no racks or panniers. Lashed to my back pack with bungee cords was a birthday gift for my young nephew: a bright yellow *Tonka* toy 'road grader,' which I had removed from its box.

Highway 46 climbs west gradually for a dozen miles or so through this part of the Santa Lucia Range, first following an old two lane County road alignment and then ascending along more recent road cuts over Black Mountain before descending steadily to the coast. The twenty two mile highway (aka Green Valley Road) has become a popular training and bicycle touring route now but in 1984, the bright yellow kid's toy strapped to my back definitely bought me some patient smiles from local truck drivers on the climb and thumbs up as they passed me speeding downhill. All things considered, it was a good jaunt to the coast – a two hour ride with a nice climb and long descent. No incidents.

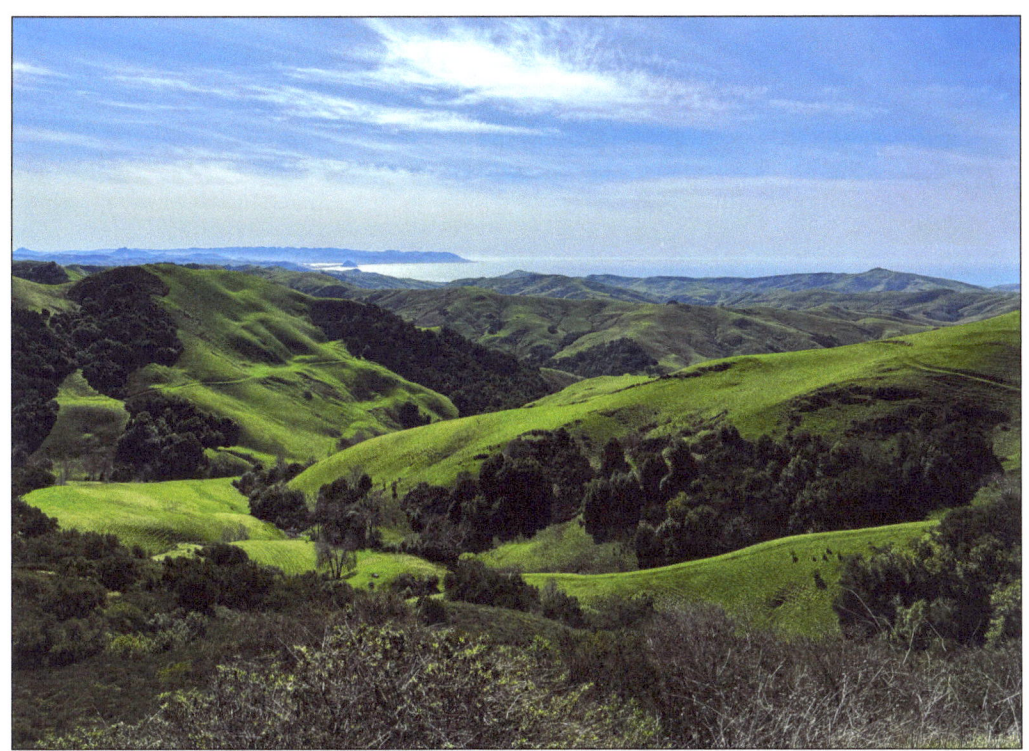

Crossing the Santa Lucia Range on Green Valley Road (Hwy 46)

Once I reached the coast another six miles of flat riding south on Highway 1 awaited. My brother lived near Villa Creek, just far enough north of Cayucos that it made sense for us to 'stay in' for an early dinner. We caught up and discussed my bike trip over pasta and wine. I gave little Tyler his four wheeled toy and repacked my gear for the eighty mile ride I had planned for the following day.

July 20th: Cayucos to Lompoc (84 mi.)

I slept well but woke up early and after chatting with my brother over coffee, fruit and cereal, I said my goodbyes and headed down the coast – south on Highway 1. Cruising through Cayucos, a layer of morning fog was hanging just low enough to obscure the horizon in the far distance. The greyness was sitting just above the nearly 600 foot high Morro Rock – about ten miles down the road. There under the dark sky was my first objective – the City of Morro Bay.

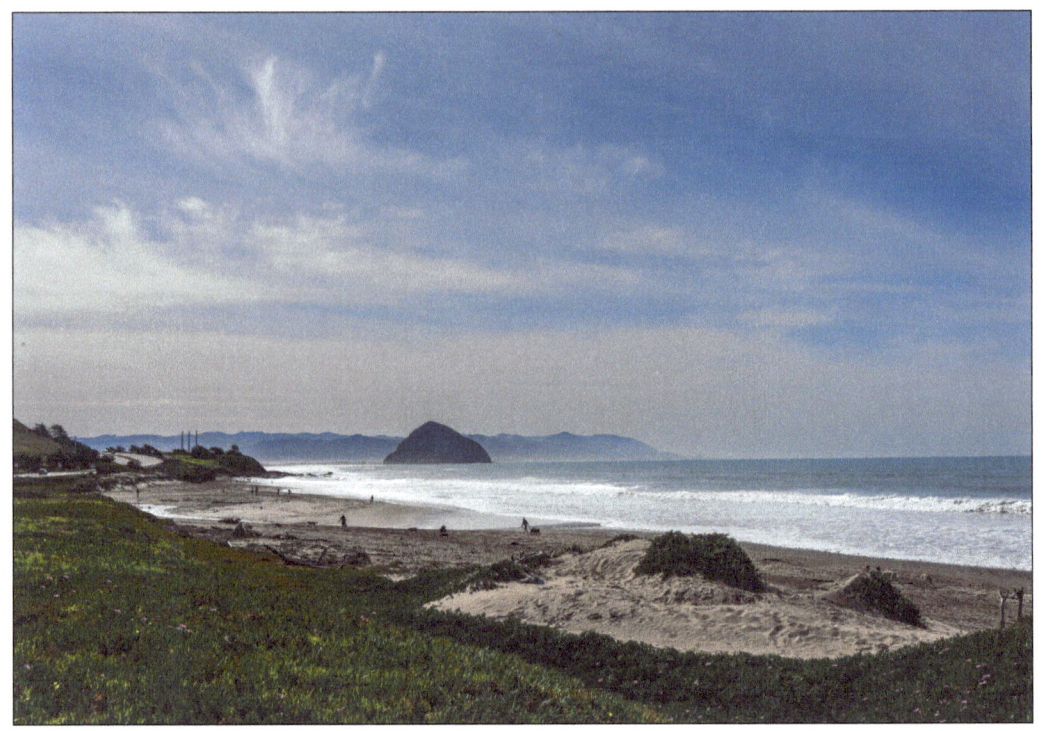

Hwy 1 view downcoast towards Morro Rock and Point Buchon

Instead of burning off, the layer of fog thickened and descended. A steady tailwind also developed as the morning progressed, propelling me at a good clip southeasterly through Morro Bay and the Los Osos Valley, along the way to Pismo Beach. On a clear day, Pismo Beach presents a long fifteen mile view downcoast. However, today the impressive 150 foot high Guadalupe Dunes to the north of Mussel Point were completely obscured. Even the nearby fifty foot high Nipomo Mesa was draped in the heavy overcast.

My inner meteorologist told me that fog and coastal clouds were being pressed all along the ridgelines ahead, guaranteeing that I would be doing some wet road riding soon. I rolled along and smiled to myself as I recalled friends asking "Why in the world would you bring a rain jacket along for a ride to southern California in July?" I rode on through Oceano and sure enough, a heavy drizzle began turning to light rain.

Across the Nipomo Mesa and into the Santa Maria Valley I rode, through the flat City of Guadalupe, then onto the rolling terrain of the valley's southern side. I had suited up with the jacket earlier but now the road was wet, car headlights and windshield wipers were on and my bike's braking action was being affected. The mid day sky grew dark, as though it was already early evening. Continuing on Highway 1, I passed through Graciosa Canyon and Harris Canyon, taking it easy in the wet conditions but with the benefit of a steady tailwind. I was making good time but gradually getting soaked.

I had ridden about thirty wet miles from Pismo Beach down Highway 1. Now in northern Santa Barbara County, I was facing the last thirteen mile leg of the day's ride. After a climb south on Highway 1 through the coastal hills to Vandenberg Air Force Base I followed the rolling roads into the City of Lompoc, where I planned to stay at my parent's house. They were traveling in Spain at the time and I already knew exactly how I'd spend my evening – first, drying and cleaning my bike, then drying and repacking my gear.

The feeling that it was early evening had continued throughout the afternoon under the heavy grey skies and steady, light rain. I stopped just before Highway 1 turns south towards Vandenberg Air Force Base and Lompoc, got off my bike – took off my backpack and jacket – then attempted to squeeze the water out of my jacket. After the third squeeze, I was convinced I'd been carrying at least a kilo of rain soaked up during the ride. I drank some water, tightened the waist strap on my rucksack and headed up the sweeping curve that immediately climbed 250 feet in three quarters of a mile over the Casmalia Hills.

The climb turned out to be unpleasant in the rain, but not horrible – it was a steep, wide, well-shouldered uphill followed by a two mile downhill into the San Antonio Valley. After descending to the San Antonio Creek bridge it was onto the day's last real climb, a two mile uphill gaining 500 feet of elevation before reaching Vandenberg's main gate on Burton Mesa. From there, it was just seven miles further east along the flat and rolling mesa before a final gradual descent into the Santa Ynez Valley and the completely flat City of Lompoc.

After riding six hours, most of it in rainy conditions, I was glad to arrive at my vacationing parent's empty house with no flat tires! I quickly got out of my wet clothes and began wiping down my bike. I was anticipating that the next morning might be a wet one and I did *not* want a single drop of water resting anywhere on my bike overnight. I made some pasta, drank a beer and gave my bike a second 'going over.' From the kitchen table I examined my *'Super Blue' Colnago* – leaning against the wall, standing clean, dry and greased. My thoroughbred was shining and ready to cover the next day's objective, a journey to Santa Barbara. I finished drying my gear, repacked my rucksack and settled in with my notebook – the next day's weather was on my mind.

July 21st: Lompoc and the Santa Ynez River (20 mi.)

Awakening to the pattering of steady rain and wind rustling in the trees was fine with me. I slept in and then spent time working on my notes. I decided to wait and see if conditions outside would let up enough to allow for reasonably comfortable riding, and around noon things did begin to clear up some, but it was another eighty miles and five hours or so to my next destination: the Ventura coast. I decided to stay another night in Lompoc and take a ride to the coast. It was just ten miles to the mouth of the Santa Ynez River via Ocean Avenue – a flat, mostly two lane county road heading directly west from downtown.

Whether or not it was the remnants of the previous day's light storm or an early afternoon sea breeze, I could feel right away that I was in for a windy one. I took off heading directly into a steady breeze blowing from the coast. It was one of those bright cloudy days, when what might ordinarily be an easy flat jaunt at times turns out to be a bunch of work. In this case it was *ten* miles of work, punching into the wind for forty five minutes.

It was work but seeing Ocean Park and the Santa Ynez river mouth was undeniably worth it. Despite the railroad trestle across lower river it's one of those rare and impressive central coast wetlands, with a well preserved and protected estuary, often full of wildlife, coupled with the often windy but inspiring 1,000 foot swath of sand dunes and beach. Sunlight reflecting on the blue ocean and spectacular central coast waves here presents a superb setting for classic 'seacoast' paintings.

I watched the numerous shorebirds in the estuary for a while from the edge of the parking lot at Ocean Park – nestled out of the wind below the trestle. I was ready to start my return when I heard the Amtrak Coast Starlight approaching. I waited

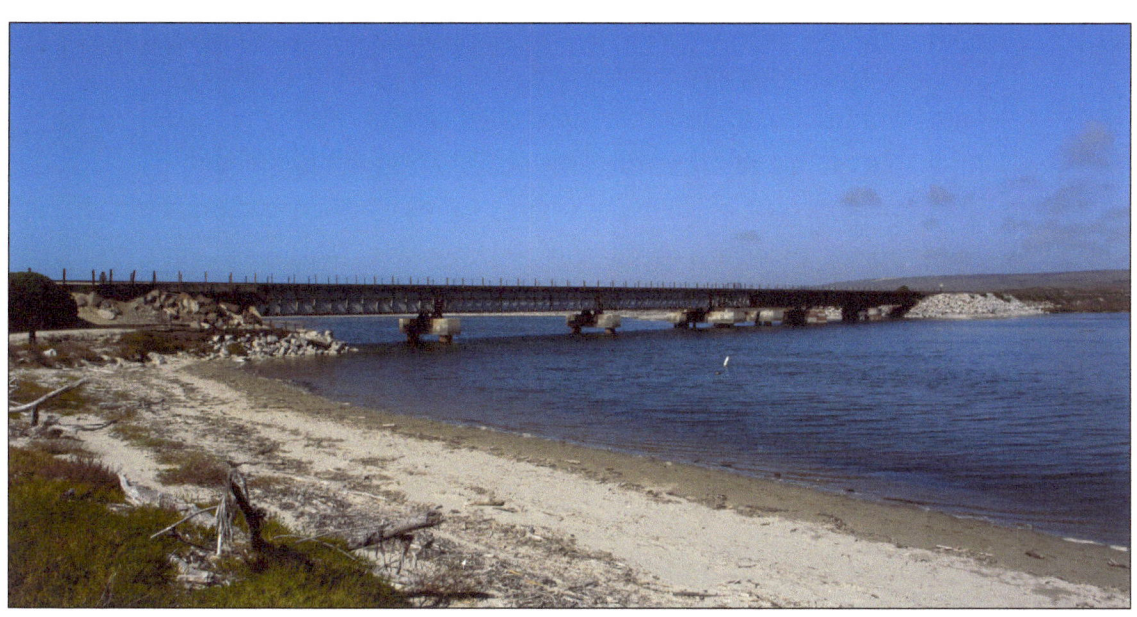

Southern Pacific railroad trestle at the Santa Ynez River mouth, northern Santa Barbara County

to see the train pass by and noticed two girls – teenagers – standing near their car giggling. As the engine passed, both of them suddenly stripped off their shirts and began jumping and dancing – screaming and laughing at the same time. *Okay,* I thought — just some good, clean adolescent fun!

Having just turned thirty, I appreciated the entertainment but was more interested in getting the other half of my ride done. It had already been more of a workout than I had planned so after taking in the views and the *flash dance* I began the return to Lompoc. *Wow!* Suddenly, I was being propelled up the slight incline by a fifteen mile an hour tailwind. It took less than half an hour to get back — a nice payback for my earlier effort while punching into the headwind.

July 23rd: Lompoc to Ventura (83 mi.)

After delaying my journey a second day, it was time to leave the Santa Ynez Valley and get moving south again. The weather forecast for the south central coast looked dry and the Ventura Coast beckoned. I planned to meet my girlfriend and stay a night at her sister's house in Ventura before riding on to *my* sister's house in western Los Angeles County. Leaving Lompoc under grey skies around 9 am wearing long pants and a jacket, I was hopeful that the day would warm up as I approached the Gaviota coast.

The ride along this next twenty mile section of Highway 1 south from Lompoc towards Las Cruces was perhaps the most enjoyable cycling of my entire adventure. Though I had been up and down this part of Highway 1 many times by car, the vantage point of my bicycle slowed things down tremendously and intensified my experience of all the sounds and pastoral scenery around me. At some point I lost track of time. I felt enveloped in the seemingly undisturbed, distinctly *Californian* landscape – highly scenic oak woodland, remote ranchland with small scale agricultural activity and virtually *no* traffic. The sky began to show patches of blue and I had a sense that this was how much of coastal California must have been in the early 19th century. I found this stretch of my ride superb.

The weather became progressively sunnier and the solitude felt perfect in this visually stunning place. It was quiet and peaceful, yet full of naturally harmonious individual sounds – of birds and insects, the wind – even the sound of my tires rolling along the road added to the chorus. The fresh coastal air smelled saturated with chemise and sage.

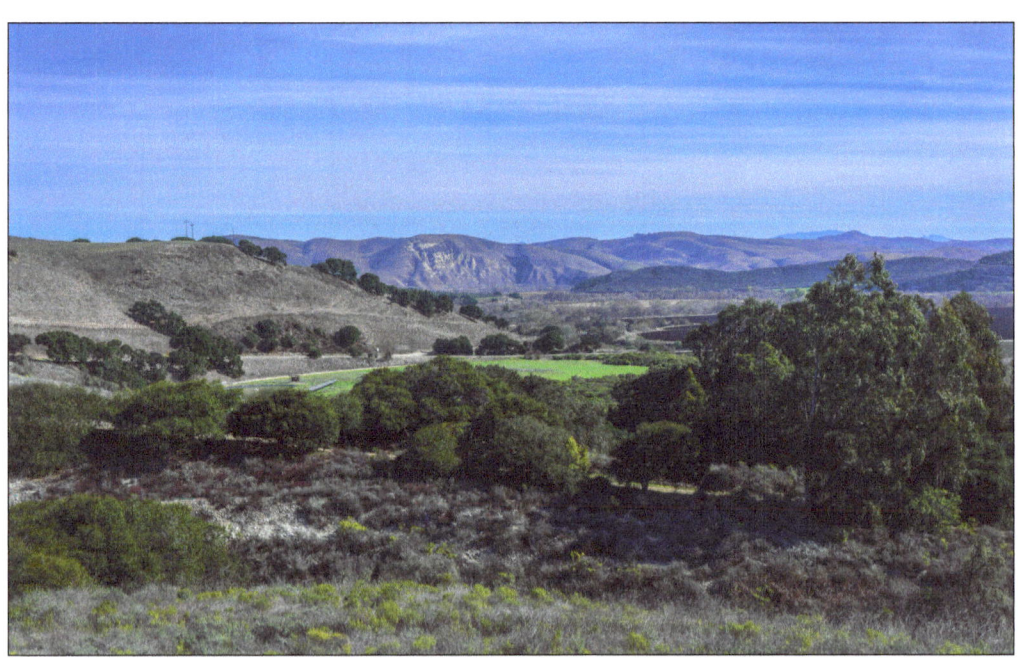

Coastal oak woodlands and ranchlands, western Santa Barbara County

As I rode on I indulged myself in the heady thinking that this was a fundamental part of why I was making this ride. I was experiencing that same feeling I'd loved when first riding a bike as a kid. I was completely independent, detached and mobile – transported and *transporting* myself. My eyes, ears, and muscles were hyper aware and ready, alert to minute changes in light, wind and road surface. I felt connected to my bike and connected to this timeless natural scene. What I experienced right then, rolling solo through rural Santa Barbara County enveloped by the pastoral scene and the aromatic landscape, has always remained one of my most memorable cycling moments.

With the light push of a westerly breeze behind me, I felt like I was pedaling effortlessly along a mild downhill gradient. I had been rolling along like this for an hour or more when the edge of the morning sun rose above the last group of low clouds ahead of me. I had covered about fifty miles in two and a half hours as I reached Gaviota Pass, where the Highway begins following the coast again. A vista point on the bluff was a gloriously sunny place for a rest stop after my sublime morning ride. I peeled off my wool riding pants and jacket.

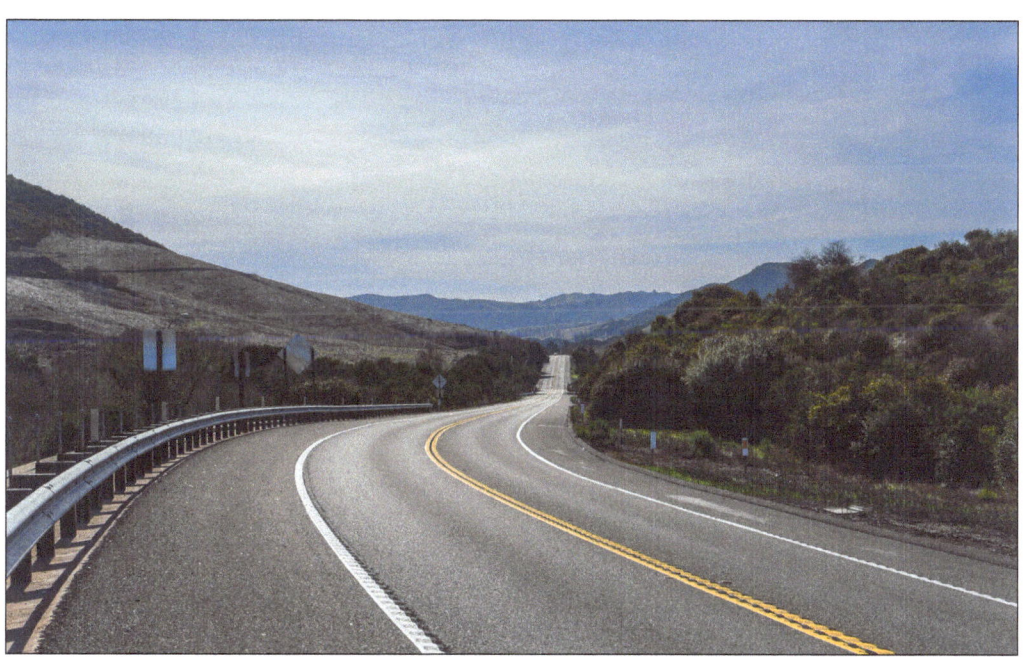

The long and winding road, Hwy 1, western Santa Barbara County

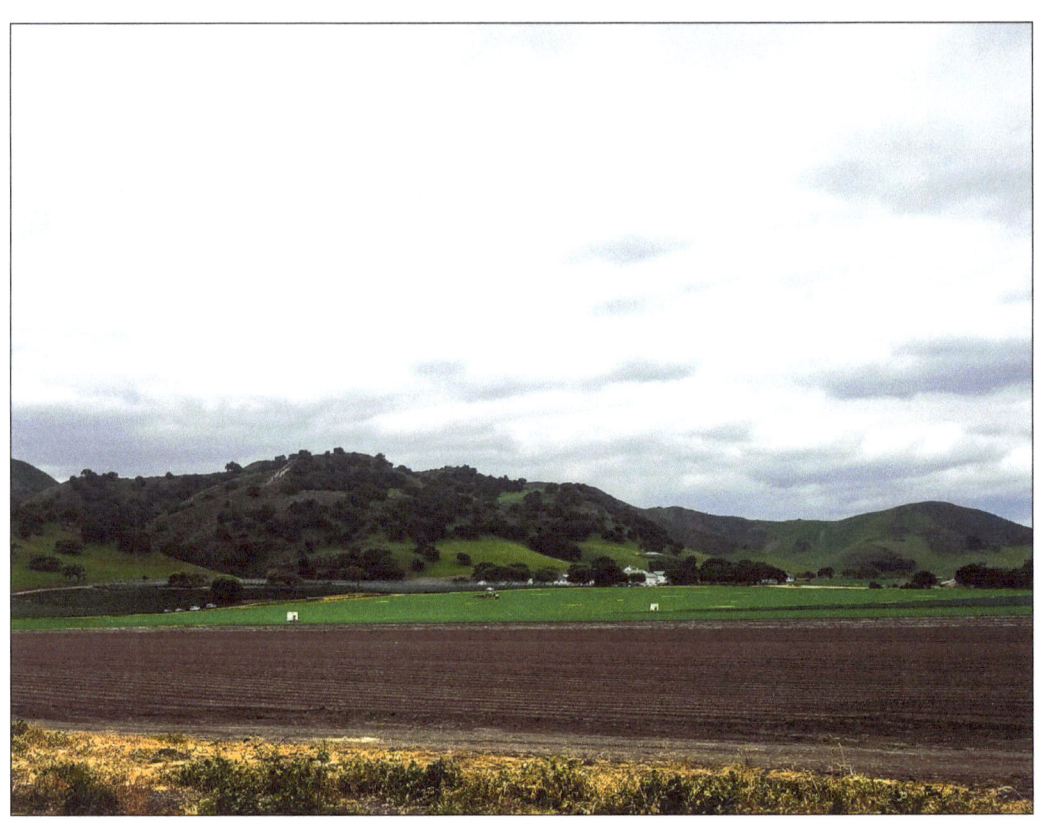

Small farms and oak woodlands, Los Alamos, western Santa Barbara County

The sunny coastal weather was great but the next part of my route – along Highway 101 from Gaviota to Goleta – was not so enjoyable. Though the highway is perched directly along the coastal bluff where views of the ocean and Santa Barbara Channel Islands can be stunning, this segment is nevertheless a federal *and* state highway. It is designed for accommodating high speed motor vehicle traffic and consequently can be tedious for touring or training cyclists – even when they're assisted by a tailwind. There are numerous large trucks that produce strong crosswinds when passing cyclists. Although the terrain is flat to rolling, the highway shoulder can also be quite narrow, especially on the bridges spanning the creeks at Arroyo Hondo, El Capitán and Refugio State Parks. Not surprisingly, this segment felt like many miles of riding alongside a noisy four lane highway.

I had planned to exit the highway at my first opportunity and follow a route riding east through Goleta along the main thoroughfares at the immediate coastline, even if it added a bit of time and distance. Once in Goleta, things changed immediately to flat, urban riding. There were lots of beach cruisers and city bikes rolling around. I made my way past Isla Vista and the University of California campus towards the harbor, then along Cabrillo Beach in the City of Santa Barbara. Eventually, my course turned inland and I proceeded through Montecito and Summerland to Carpinteria, where the shoulder of the Coast Highway beckoned again. My day's last segment would lead me into Ventura County.

Cyclists are treated to stunning views as they ride down the old Rincon Highway along the coast between Carpinteria and Ventura – especially now in 2024. Unlike Gaviota, there is a Class 1 bike lane here, physically separated from the freeway lanes. In 1984, however, the bike lane hadn't yet been built – my only option was riding along the highway shoulder. Once again, I was rolling along the bluff above the surf – with the sun, a tailwind –and truck traffic. After ten miles I was glad to be done for the day – I exited the Coast Highway and cruised into downtown Ventura.

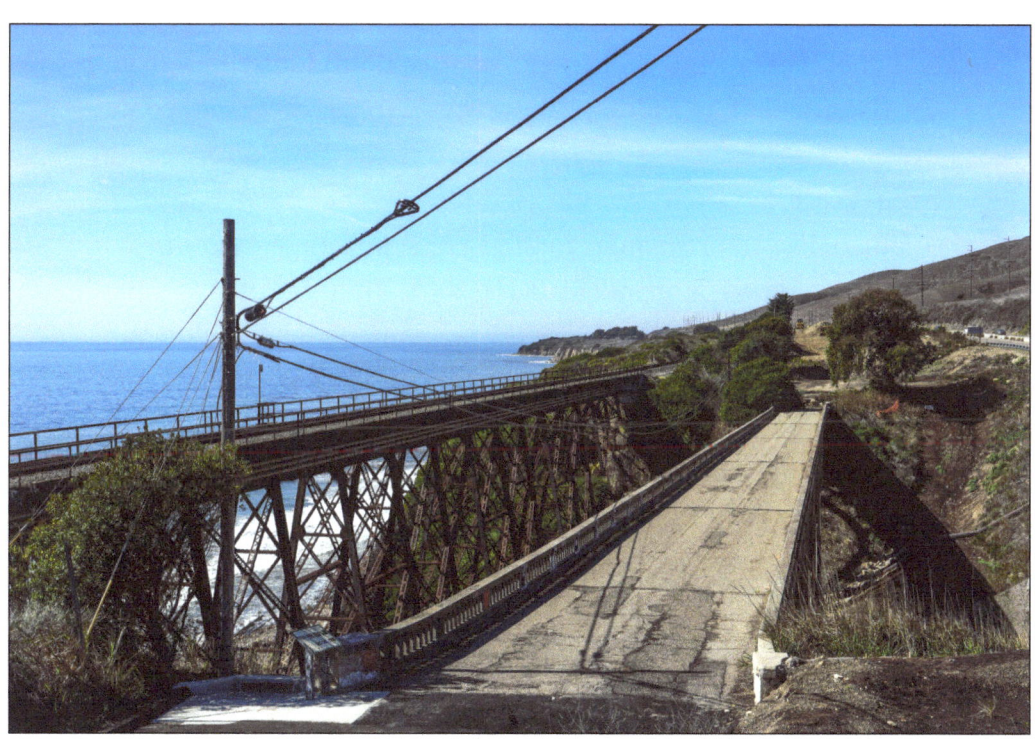

Southern Pacific railroad trestle (1900) and old Hwy 101 bridge (1919) at Arroyo Hondo, western Santa Barbara County

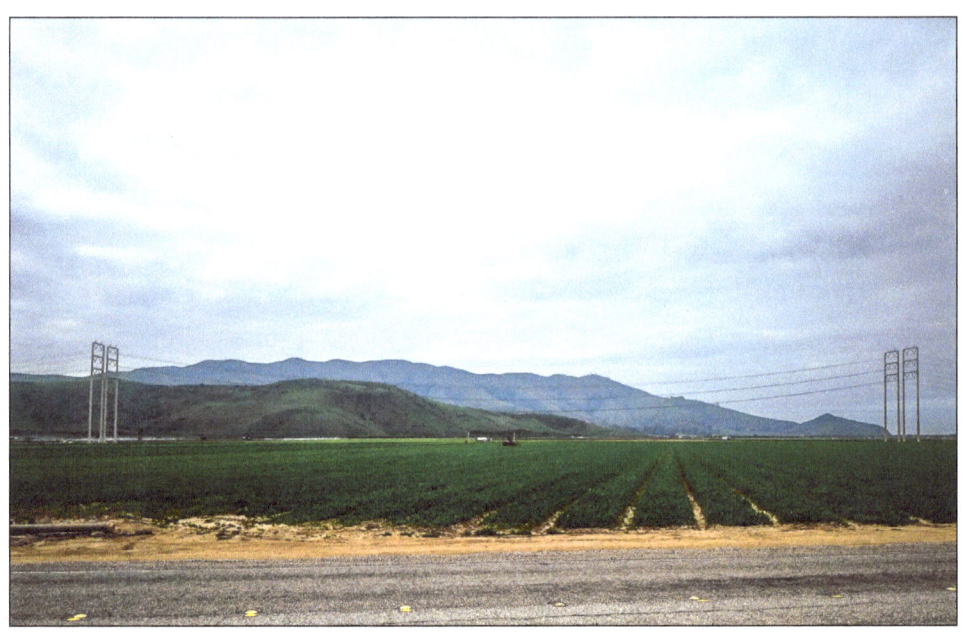

The Oxnard Plain – intensive agriculture, beckoning mountains... and rough roads

July 24th: Ventura to Agoura (45 mi.)

Another bright and sunny day dawned and I got a late morning start across the perfectly flat Oxnard plain towards the rugged terrain of the Santa Monica Mountains. My first objective was the County road that traverses this 1,500 foot climb from the Oxnard Plain to Hidden Valley. The average 6% grade would present a hot and steep ride, but was also the most direct route from Ventura to my next destination – my sister's house in Agoura – less than 50 miles to the east, in Los Angeles County.

This ride was a 'grind' from the start. After my late morning rollout I got caught in mid day traffic, immediately. The terrain was mild but city traffic through Oxnard and Port Hueneme was not. Rough pavement, narrow shoulders and short bridges seemed to be everywhere. There were detours, speeding cars, slow moving farm vehicles and equipment on the road, chemical odors – and *no tailwind.* The air temperature was already reaching 80°F (27°C) and I was dripping sweat. It had taken nearly two hours to work my way thirty miles through both cities and across the intensively farmed flatlands to the base of the climb. From there I began what would be a steep, difficult three mile ascent on Potrero Road in the open sun and maximum afternoon heat. I shifted to my lowest gear and started making my way up the grade, intent on preserving my water.

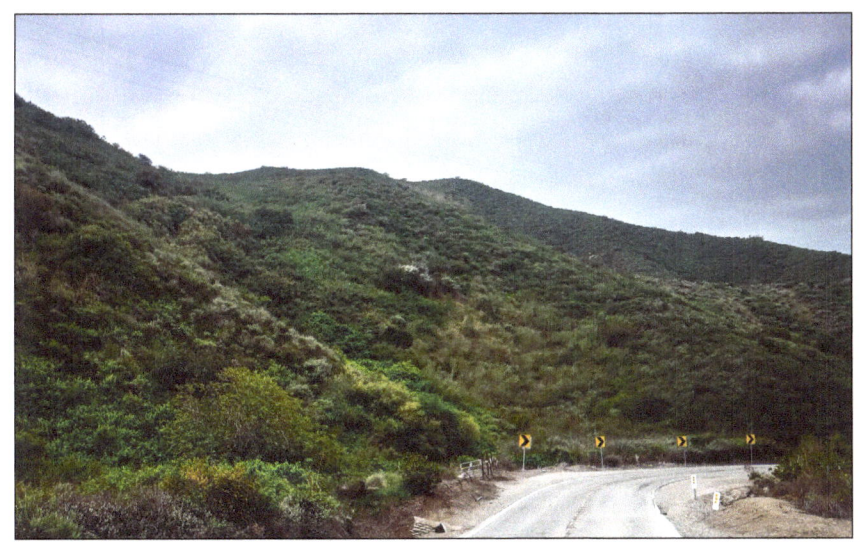

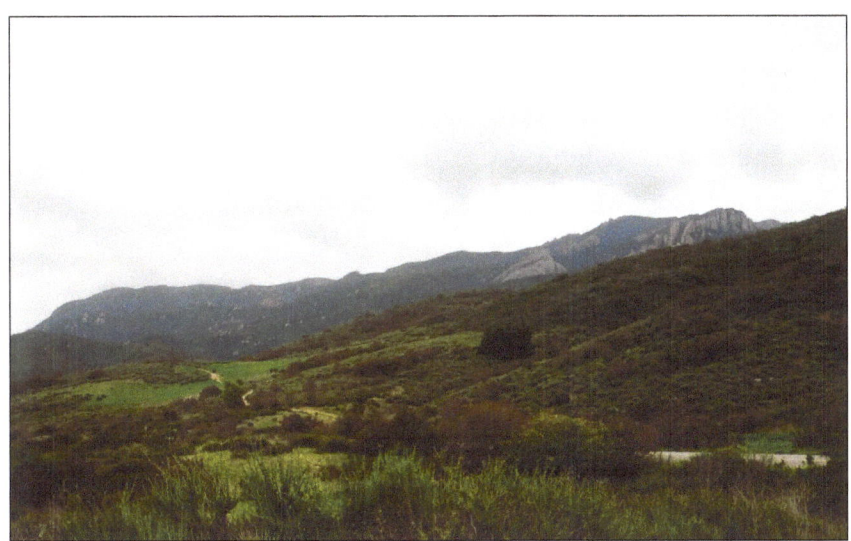

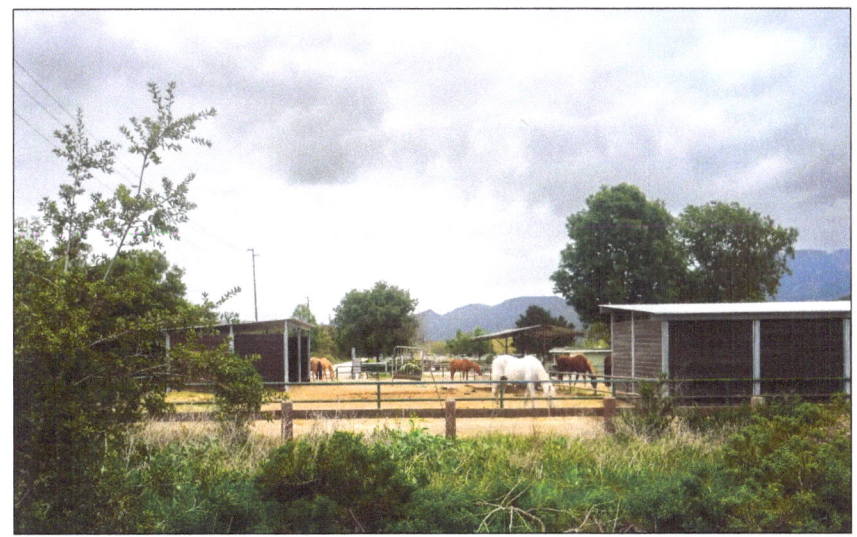

Beginning the ascent on Potrero Road (u), Split Rock, sandstone peaks in the western Santa Monica Mountains (m), Rancho Potrero Community Stables (l), Ventura County

After climbing for thirty minutes I'd covered about three miles, conquered several 15% inclines and reached the first plateaus of the Santa Monica Mountains at Dos Vientos Ranch, almost 1000 feet above sea level and downtown Ventura, where I began. Another eight miles and 500 more feet of climbing brought me to Hidden Valley, where exclusive thoroughbred farms abound, adding to the rugged backdrop of sculpted sandstone peaks in the nearby Santa Monica Mountains. There were llamas, alpacas and beautiful purebred horses – whitewashed wooden fence rails and irrigated turf. As I rode slowly by, some of the curious quadrupeds approached their fences for a closer look at me but nothing could take my mind off the heat of the afternoon.

Climbing over 1500 feet in the mid day sun had exhausted me. My *second* water bottle was nearly empty! I rode another mile and a half, climbing the last 100 feet of the day before descending to Westlake Village, where I stopped to fill up both water bottles and put another dab of sunscreen on my nose. In the shade of a school roof awning was a large thermometer reading 108° F (42° C). My watch read 3:30.

I continued on Agoura Road to about a mile from my sister's house and decided to find a phone and let her know I was getting close to her place. Of course, there were no cell phones in 1984... she was waiting for me to call. She was ready to head to the store and we agreed I would stay where I was while she shopped before picking me up in her van.

I found a shady spot and worked on my notes. Soon she arrived with a van full of groceries and her two young boys – with room to spare for one overheated cyclist and his machine. We headed off to Agoura Hills where a pool and Jacuzzi awaited

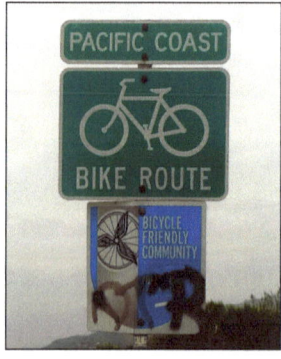

The Pacific Coast Bike Route, Ventura County

my excited nephews and me. It's safe to say neither had ever seen this much intensity related to cycling. They knew that I would visit and see the Olympic cycling events but they had never smelled someone who had been riding for 3 hours or seen dried streaks of salty sweat on a cycling jersey.

I could hear the boys splashing in the pool and discussing their bikes as I showered in the guest room next to my sister's back yard. The time was approaching 5 pm and I headed for the hot tub, intent on half an hour of hydro treatment before dinner.

The Jacuzzi gave me time to reflect on my journey thus far. This was the sixth night and everything had gone exceptionally well. I felt mentally transported back to some unique moments. The Tonka truck smiles, the downhill miles, the rain, the terrain, the train engineer's 'girlie show,' the sun and solitude. The fifty mile segment of Highway 1 between Lompoc to Gaviota struck me as the high point – the palettes of color, sounds and smells, arriving at the sunny coast and blue ocean. Even climbing up the western edge of the Santa Monica Mountains in the afternoon heat was quite a feat. So far, my trip had been *Mission: Accomplished.* Next on the agenda would be attending the opening ceremonies of the XXIII Olympiad at the Los Angeles Coliseum.

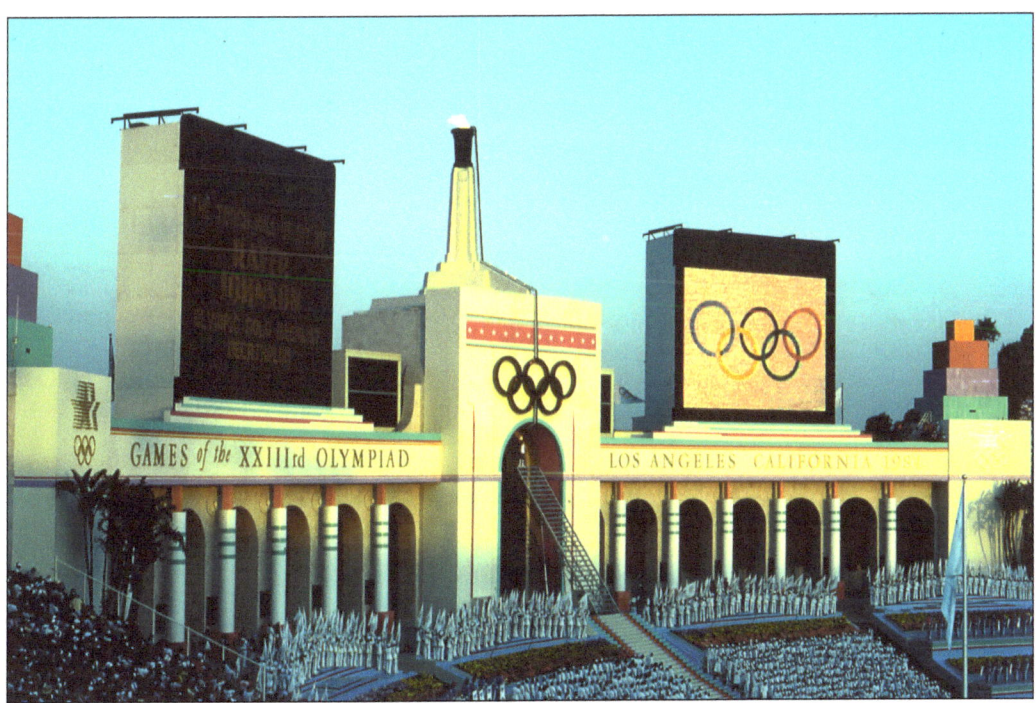

Lighting the Olympic Torch at the opening ceremonies of the XXIII Olympiad, Los Angeles Coliseum, July 28, 1984

I race to win – not to please people

– BERNARD HINAULT
French professional cycling hero and five time winner of the *Tour de France*

Chased Down and Dropped by the Swiss Olympic Team (1984)

Having overnighted in Malibu, I awoke at seven and suited up for a sunny and bright morning ride up the coast. I freewheeled down to Pacific Coast Highway and headed west paralleling the shore. It was 'PCH' at its best – rolling along the wide, well paved shoulder with no traffic – early on a Saturday. As the sun rose behind me the layered sandstone bluffs ahead were lit up in shades of red, yellow-brown and fiery gold. Jagged and dark, the profile of Anacapa Island broke the flat line of the ocean's horizon. My destination was in view. Point Mugu abruptly rose 170 feet at the coastline about fifteen miles away in Ventura County.

After an hour or so I arrived at Point Mugu. I turned into the vista point parking area next to the point itself where got off the bike, stretched and watched the waves. There was no fog and jets were continuously taking off from the Naval Air Station at nearby Mugu Lagoon. I took a few pictures but the sky was already a hazy flightpath. The numerous shorebirds, pelicans and gulls seemed completely indifferent to the engine noise and exhaust. After checking my tires I was ready to begin my return downcoast to Malibu. There was no breeze or tailwind.

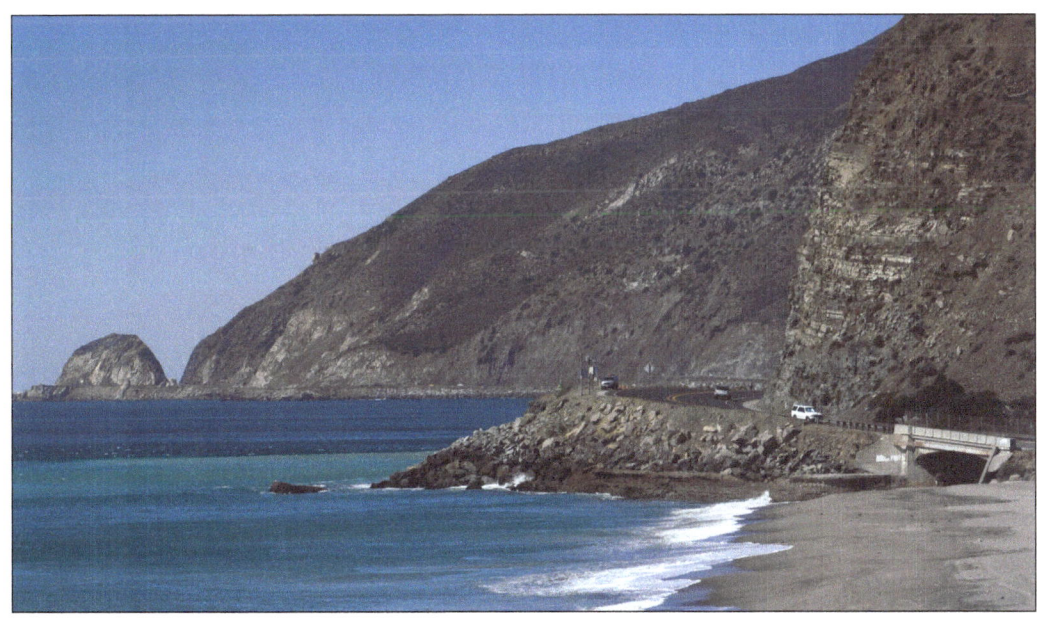

Point Mugu and Pacific Coast Highway (Highway 1), Ventura County

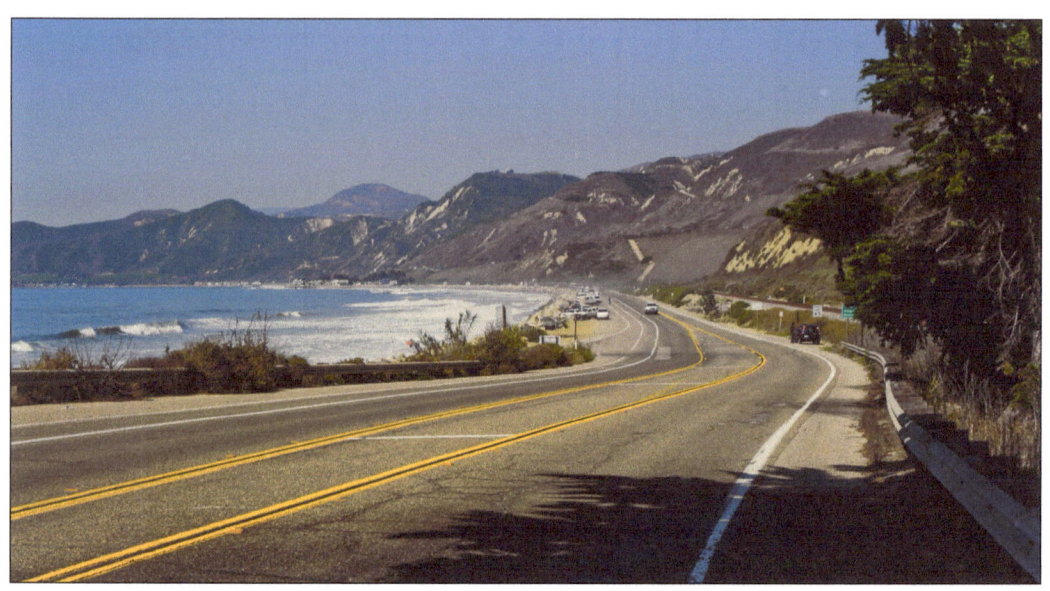
Pacific Coast Highway (Highway 1), Ventura County

The air remained calm and stagnant but cleared as I got further from Point Mugu. I was happy to be smelling the salty ocean again – not aviation fuel! Southbound auto traffic was increasing. Though riding along the Ventura/Malibu coastline was markedly different than traversing coastal ranchland in Santa Barbara County, I was enjoying myself. This particular July morning, Malibu's mostly south facing coastline was sunny and beautiful – less remote than its upcoast counterpart but every bit as exceptional. The morning sunlight reflecting on the breaking waves looked dazzling. I was transported by the sounds of the surf and gulls in concert with the rhythmic humming of my wheels and drive train. That feeling of 'bicycle bliss' began overtaking me.

Well… that wasn't the only thing overtaking me. My state of seemingly effortless motion and detachment was over when I heard the mechanical sound of derailleurs shifting. I knew more than one bike was approaching from behind me. With a quick glance back I saw a team of riders wearing red and white jerseys about to catch me. A four door American sedan was following closely behind their group.

I was rolling along quite briskly but the group passed me with little effort. I could see their jerseys. I'd been caught by the men's Olympic cycling team from Switzerland – out for a training ride up the coast. I figured that they had started earlier and ridden farther north than I had. Now on their way back, they had passed me at close to 25 miles an hour. A couple of the riders nodded as they cruised by on my left but their intent was clear: keep the pace high and get past the guy on the *Colnago*. We were about five miles west of town.

Riding seriously, you learn about slipstreams and drafting. My friends and I had learned long before to 'take a pull' in front and then switch positions, tucking in behind the other rider for a respite, especially in a headwind. I decided I would stay close and take advantage of the pulling effect of this pack of fit elite athletes in front of me. I changed gears and upped my pace to mark the rear rider. For a moment, it felt effortless – like flying.

I had no sense that I was interfering with the team's training but the sedan immediately sped up to the head of the pace line for a moment and then gradually dropped back to the rear of their group. I noticed the front seat passenger was glaring at me about the same time I felt the speed of the group pick up significantly. It was clear that I wasn't supposed to be hanging on to these guys – they now had instructions to drop me.

And drop me they did, cranking up the cadence to an intense high level, knowing that I wasn't going to jump into their line. They pulled away from me on the first sustained rise and resumed their usual training regimen, disappearing over the rolling terrain that lay up ahead. Of course, at the time, none of us knew that eight days later on August 5th four members of this Swiss Olympic cycling team would win a silver medal in the 100 kilometer team time trial, finishing in just over two hours – four minutes behind an Italian team that took the gold medal and eight seconds ahead of the USA's team that took bronze.

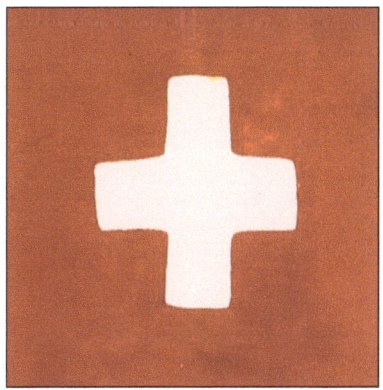

Detail from a Swiss National Cycling Team jersey

*Under the best circumstances the experience
of cycling is more about the ride
than the destination*

– JVC

Road and Track Cycling at the XXIII Olympiad (1984)

July 29th: The Road Races in Mission Viejo

Attending the Olympic Road Races was free but *not* easy. Maybe part of it was easy – the first part – getting to the race course from Huntington Beach. The mid morning skies were clear and the temperature was perfect for cycling on the bike path at the coast and along the shore of Newport Bay. Nevertheless, I knew that it would eventually be a 'scorcher.' As my girlfriend and I made our way inland through Irvine and El Toro to Mission Viejo it felt hot and dry – the late morning temperature was approaching 85°F (30°C). For a couple of northern Californians, it was sweltering heat – when sweat evaporates and you feel 'baked' no matter how much liquid you drink.

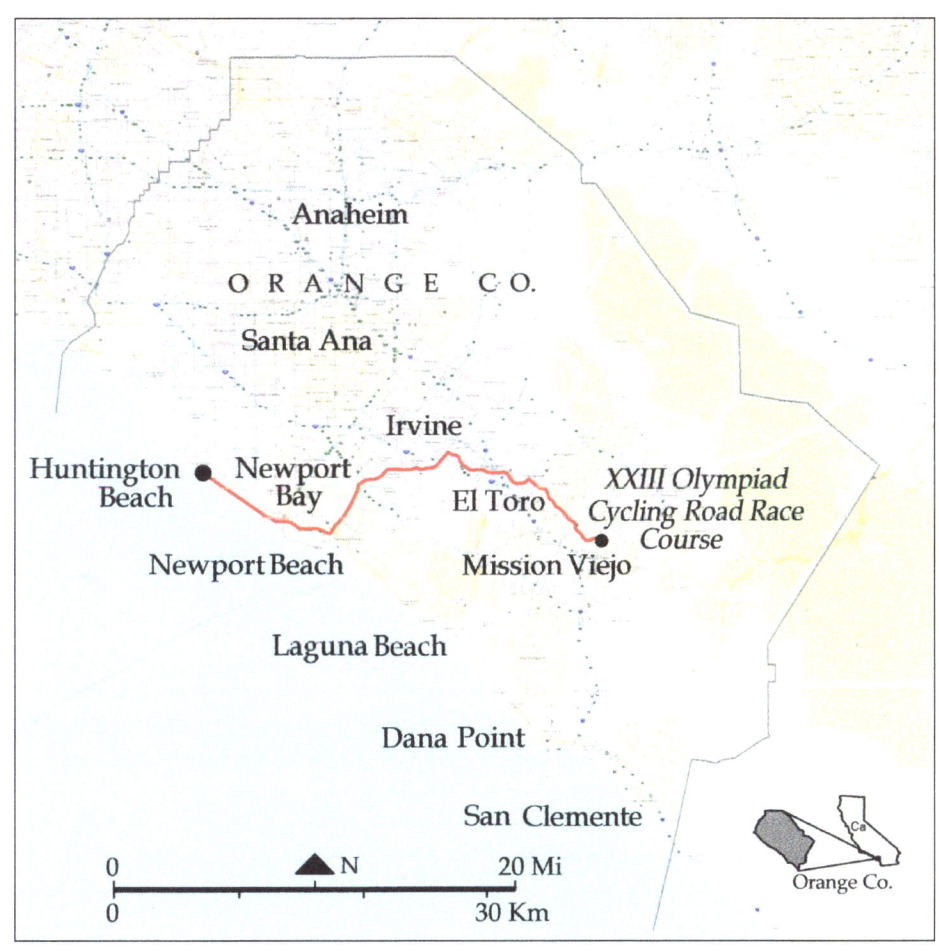

Cycling route to the 1984 Olympic Road Races in Orange County

Fortunately, our early arrival allowed us to take possession of a shady spot along O'Neill Road next to a retaining wall near the finish line.[7] The shadow cast by the wall was quickly shrinking as the sun rose steadily along its high summertime arc. An estimated 100,000 spectators lining the ten mile course were about to get a serious sunbath.

Despite needing hats, sunscreen and lots of water, watching the 49 mile women's and 118 mile long men's circuit races among a sea of energized cycling fans was undeniably exciting. There was huge anticipation about the *first ever* women's Olympic road race *and* the possibility that members of the USA cycling teams might medal for the first time in 72 years.[8] The top USA cyclists were enduring a lot of pressure, scrutiny and expectations leading up to the games. The press had played up rivalries between teammates and covered the latest doping cases. Now the athletes would face each other in 90°F (33°C) heat on a 9.8 mile course that included freshly paved blacktop and 1,590 feet of climbing.

The women's race was five laps and the men's race twelve. Predictably, both races seemed to unfold in the final two laps. The two hour long women's race saw six women break away and gain a two minute lead on the pack with about one lap to go before the final sprint. In the end, Rebecca Twigg seemed to have the advantage but moved slightly off a straight line as Connie Carpenter-Phinney edged out her teammate and rival by less than half a wheel in the burst for the finish line. In doing so, she became the first USA cyclist to medal since the 1912 Games and had won the first ever *gold* medal for a cyclist from the USA. Rebecca Twigg received the silver medal.

The men's race began at 1 pm and after completing 10 laps in the extreme heat there were six riders in a breakaway group, including USA favorite Davis Phinney, his teammate Alexi Grewal and Canadian Steve Bauer. Grewal attacked the breakaway and had gained a twenty second advantage with just one lap to go, then suddenly faltered on the climb up Vista del Lago and was caught by Canadian Steve Bauer. The two stayed together and surged ahead of Davis Phinney and the other chasers, then contested a classic two man sprint finish with Alexi Grewal

---
7. Subsequently renamed Olympiad Road.
8. The Soviet Union and Eastern Bloc countries boycotted the 1984 Olympics.

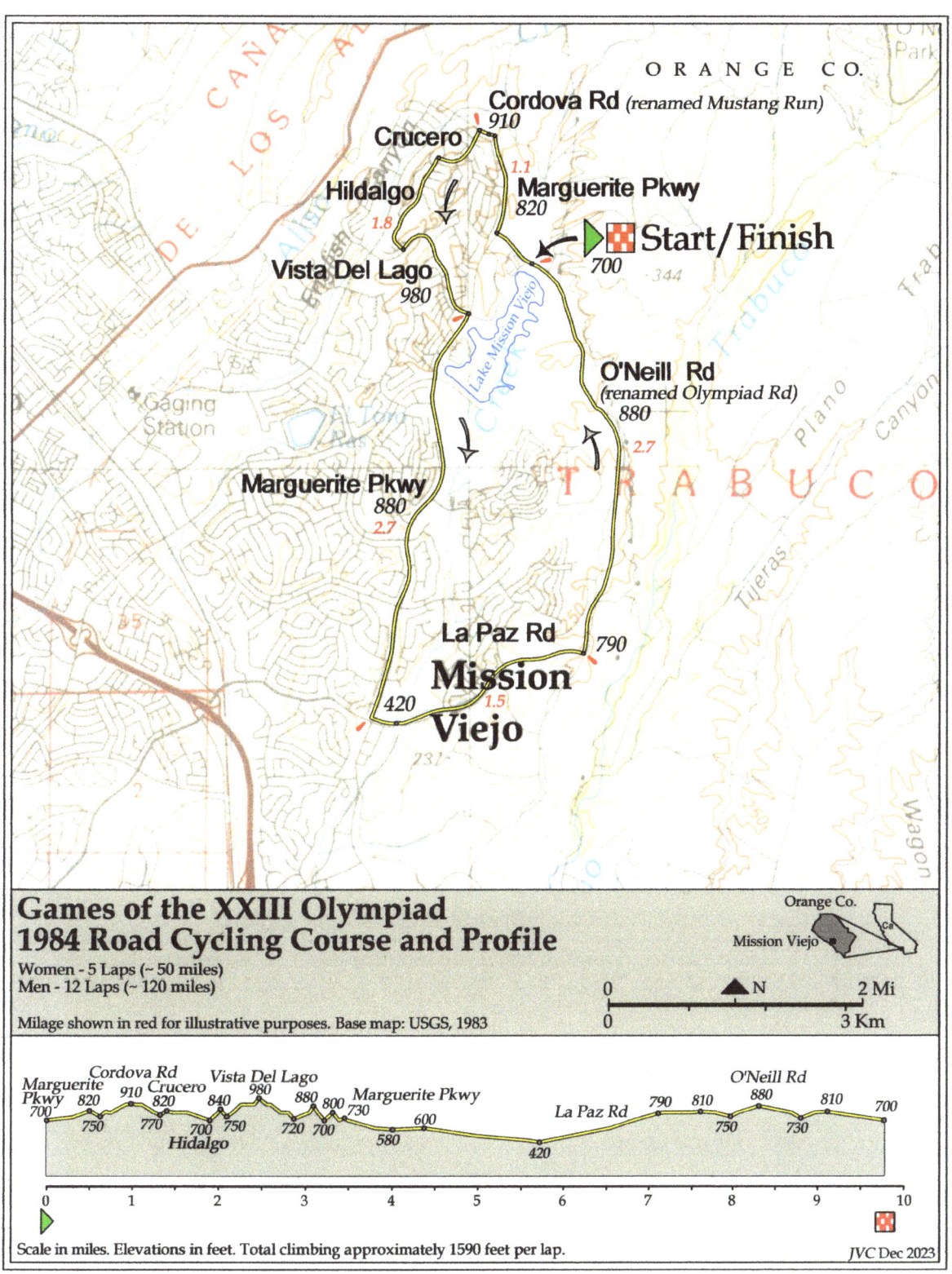

pulling away to win the gold medal by about a bike length. He had won a third Olympic cycling medal for the USA! The roasted crowd of thousands lining the course loved it – chanting "U—S—A" as they waited to see their two wheeled heroes pass by once more along Marguerite Parkway. *Fifty five* of the racers did not finish the men's event that day. By late afternoon, vendors were selling bottles of water for two dollars each!

The ride back to Huntington Beach turned out to be more trying than the afternoon heat. It was near 6 pm when the racing ended. By the time we began the sinuous route west the sun had nearly dropped below the coastal hills ahead of us. Twilight brought with it blinding automobile headlights and dark stretches of unlit bike path where our likewise unlit bicycles carried us slowly up the coast past Newport Beach. Bringing along my bicycle light simply had not crossed my mind that morning.

Once safely back, all I could think about was how exciting the day had been from one end to the other. Amazingly, not one but *three* USA cyclists had medaled for the first time since 1912. It was the USA's first ever gold in the men's road race. The USA had taken gold and silver medals in the first ever women's road race. The fact that Davis Phinney had been the favorite for the United States and that Alexi Grewal had been suspended literally days before made Grewal's win even more amazing.[9] First banned, then reinstated and allowed to race, he responded by defeating all rivals, covering the 118 mile course in under five hours.

August 1st and 3rd: Track Events at Dominguez Hills

By 1984, the 7 Eleven Corporation had been sponsoring a bicycle racing team for several years and provided the funding for the construction of the outdoor Olympic velodrome on the campus of the California State University at Dominguez Hills in Carson, California. The velodrome events of the XXIII Olympiad were some of the most popular and I had purchased tickets early. I was excited to watch the 4,000 meter Pursuit and the Match Sprint races, where, due in part to a boycott of the Olympic Games by the Soviet Union and East Germany, the USA racers were dominant and took *five* medals in these two events.

---

9. Grewal had been suspended from the team on July 18th after a positive doping test result and was reinstated on the team three days later.

The next three days was full of track cycling excitement. Watching the USA rider Steve Hegg dominate the 4,000 meter Pursuit – eventually taking the gold in the finals – while his teammate Leonard Harvey Nitz grabbed the bronze medal, was superb. Mark Gorski and Nelson Vails also provided a winning one-two combination for the USA in the Match Sprint events. These four and the Team Pursuit squad contributed to some patriotic victory lap scenes, with the racers in their blue skinsuits, white-starred and red-striped – waving miniature USA flags. Gorski rode with his young son perched on the handlebars.

An interesting side note about the 1984 cycling events was that they took place in an era when 'blood packing' (using transfusions to increase the amount of red blood cells in one's blood) and the use of other performance enhancing drugs were considered legitimate components of an elite cyclist's training program. After the 1984 Olympic Games a third of the USA cycling team admitted receiving transfusions – which was done openly and had not yet been prohibited. It wasn't until *1985* that blood 'doping' was banned in the United States – though no test was yet available to detect it. Interestingly, a mere year later when the Soviet Union and East Germany track racers participated at the 1986 World Cycling Championships held in Colorado, most of the elite USA racers were eliminated early, never reaching even the quarter final events in the Match Sprint *or* the 4,000 meter Pursuit.

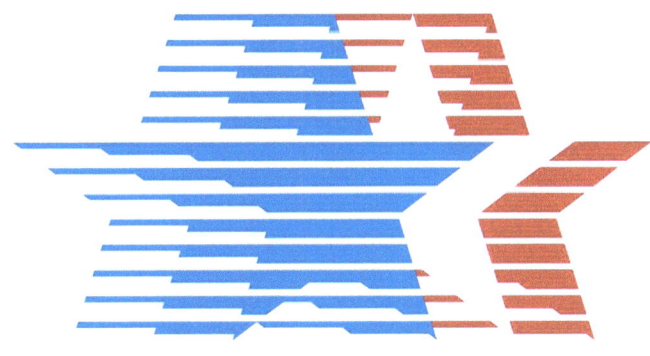

Games of the XXIIIrd Olympiad Los Angeles 1984

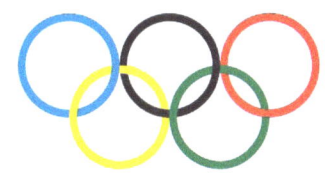

It was like a long training ride[10]

– GREG LEMOND
   American professional cycling hero and three time *Tour de France* winner

---

10. Describing the bike race part of 1985's *World's Toughest Triathlon* – which included 9,000 feet of climbing and 120 high elevation miles in the Sierra Nevada, south of Lake Tahoe.

The *World's Toughest Triathlon* or Poppin' the Hip (1985)

In early August of 1984 I returned from my bicycling adventure of riding along California's central coast to Los Angeles and seeing the cycling events at the Summer Olympics.[11] I was inspired and superbly fit and immediately began extending the duration of my training rides. Living in Marin County I could always find hilly terrain and realized that, for me, *time* spent on the bike was as important as terrain or distance. In other words, being fit enough to manage a four or five hour ride was a better gauge of my conditioning than simply having climbed a steep peak or completed a century.[12] Out of necessity I had become a decent climber for someone over six feet tall and during rides with some of my sportsman friends I began to dream and scheme about participating in a timed long distance cycling event.

Many of my highly competitive friends were becoming aware of the new sport of triathlon due to television coverage of the *Hawaii Ironman* and one of them found out about a California race dubbed The *World's Toughest Triathlon* – its 2nd edition to be held at South Lake Tahoe that September. Several of us braved the Labor Day holiday traffic and drove up to the Lake in order to watch the 1984 race, which consisted of a 2.4 mile swim in the lake, followed by a 120 mile bike race including about 9,000 feet of climbing over Sierra Nevada passes, then finishing with a *26.7* mile marathon, much of it on fire roads and trails. High elevations and mountain weather were also factors.

Scott Molina, a professional triathlete in his mid twenties, won the ironman division that year. With a time just over 10 hours and 29 minutes, he finished *42* minutes ahead of second place winner Barry Makarewicz and broke the course record by an hour and a half!

My friends and I decided right away that we wanted to participate in the 3rd edition the following year. Three of us in our early thirties – fellow high school mates Noel Laverty, Shawn

---

11. During the span of one week, I was able to attend the opening ceremonies and a number of road and track cycling events.
12. A century is a 100 mile ride. A metric century is a 100 kilometer ride (62.0 miles).

Ridley and I – signed up for the team relay category as soon as the 1985 event was confirmed. Noel would swim, I would bike, and Shawn would run. *Team JNS* was formed and I continued my training all through fall and winter. The top ten male cyclists had finished the 1984 course in seven hours or less. The top five women cyclists all finished in less than seven and a half hours!

Another great cycling year unfolded for me in 1985, right up until the fateful end of that year's edition of this triathlon, at 4 pm on Saturday, September 7th. All that year, my life revolved around cycling, training and following races. I studied topographic maps of the triathlon's bike course. Riding with others or alone, climbing to Pantoll Station or Mount Tamalpais became part of my routine. Regular training for the race provided a perfect reason to spend more time on the bike. As Spring progressed I began weaving in 100 mile club rides with complete strangers. I enjoyed my usual long steady rides with cycling comrades but spent the majority of time training solo. By Summer's end I was feeling strong and ready to meet the challenge of competing in the *World's Toughest Triathlon.*

As September approached, I received word that our friend Frank Varvaro had arranged lodging for us at Tahoe Keys. *Team JNS* was to occupy a large house located right on the lake – available for the entire week prior to the race.

My girlfriend and I arrived at the Lake early in the week before the race, intending to have a few days for acclimation to the mountain air. The next day I decided we would drive out to Topaz Lake with my bike so that I could ride the climb to Monitor Pass along Highway 89. I'd ridden *around* Lake Tahoe before but wanted to know what it felt like to push myself over an 8,300 foot high Sierra Nevada pass. Predictably, it turned out to be tough, steady work in my *Colnago*'s 'not so low' lowest gear but the twelve mile climb with over 3,000 feet of elevation gain presented some remarkable views east towards Nevada's basin and range lands. The stunning scenery was motivation to keep plowing uphill – along with my expectations of a fast descent to Markleeville… *and a well earned late lunch!*

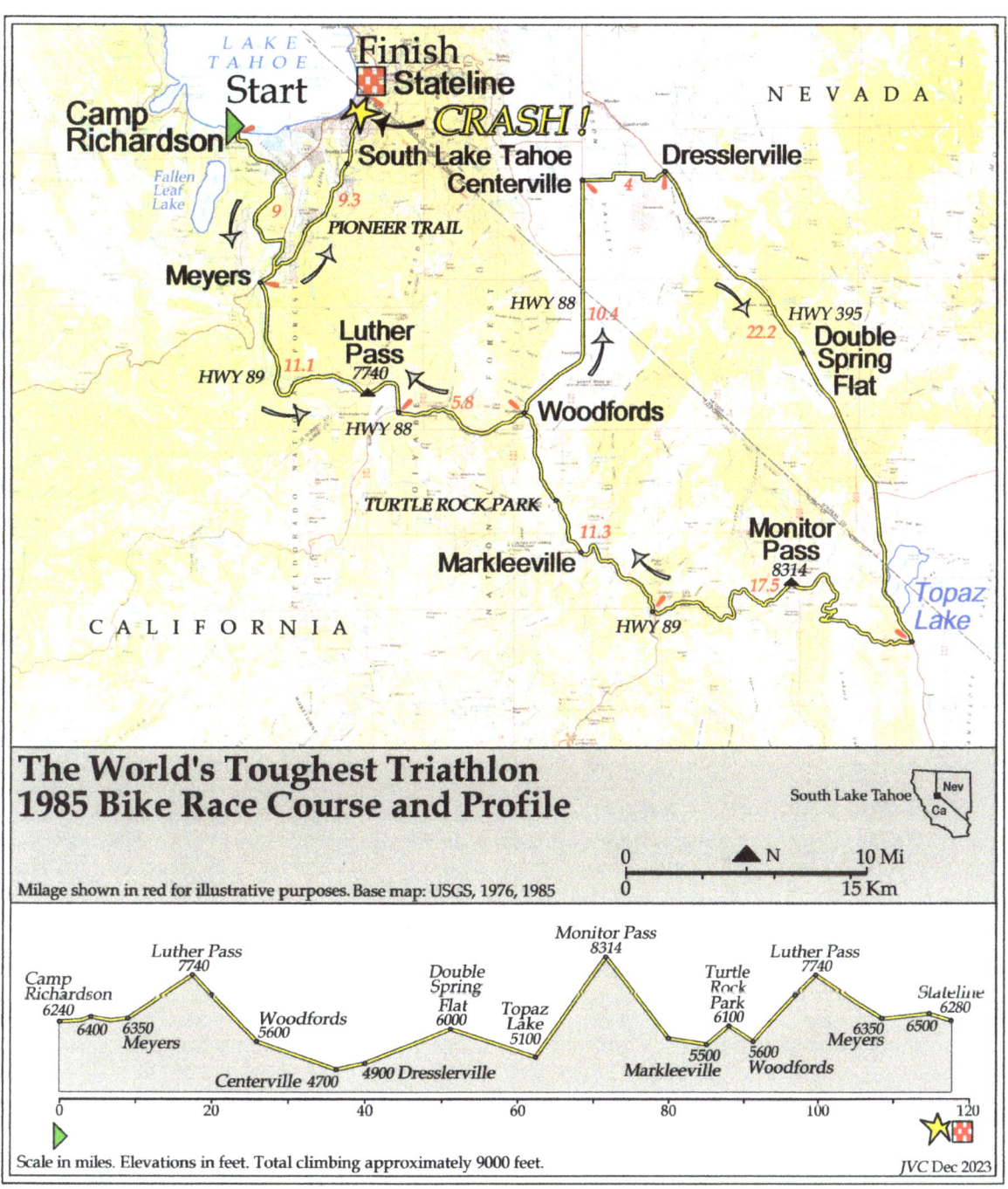

At the crest of Monitor Pass, afternoon thundershowers commenced, making my steep downhill nerve wracking and dangerous. The slippery, metal 'cattle guards' crossing the road at several locations also made it difficult to maintain any momentum. There was absolutely no reason to take risks and I chose to simply roll down steadily – hands ready on the brakes – controlling my pace. I arrived in town and met my girlfriend at the Cutthroat Saloon, where dry clothes, a 'French Dip' roast beef sandwich and a dark beer made it all seem worth worthwhile.

Two days later I decided to do my final race preparation by climbing Luther Pass from both directions. I rode out from Tahoe Keys early enough to miss the afternoon thunderstorms but got caught in a stream of RVs and trucks bound for Lake Tahoe on my way back. Luther Pass is a shorter climb with half the elevation gain of its giant neighbor – Monitor Pass – but it is still steep and features much more regular vehicle traffic.

This section of Highway 89 is a main route in and out of South Lake Tahoe. I soon found myself alongside a line of slow moving vehicles – forced to use my brakes on the descent. It was a lesson in how to avoid RVs and logging trucks weaving in and out of the 'bike lane' as they maneuvered down the two lane sections of highway leading to Meyers. The following day at the pre-race registration we were informed that the race course would be heavily signed and all cattle guards covered. Saturday's weather was expected to remain the same.

I can't recall whether or not I slept well Friday night but, regardless, I was up at dawn on Saturday and ready to go. Earlier in the week the news had come out that the top American pro cyclist Greg LeMond would compete in the relay division, racing the bike leg for *Team Kahlua*. I wanted to get to Camp Richardson and satisfy my curiosity, not so much about his celebrity status – I couldn't stop wondering about his choice of gearing! I knew his bike would be somewhere in the swim/bike transition area.

At 23, LeMond was a rising star in pro cycling and had already been road race winner in the 1983 World Cycling Championships.[13] In July of 1985, he had become the first American to place 2nd in

---

13. Acknowledged as one of professional cycling's all time top champions, Greg LeMond would go on to win the *Tour de France* in 1986, 1989, and 1990.

the most prestigious of all professional bicycle races, Le *Tour de France*. In August he had taken 2nd in the road race at the World Cycling Championships. The media had created some drama about whether LeMond would better 1984 Ironman winner Scott Molina's 'split time' for the bike leg. Molina had set a new course record at 5:39:21 the previous year, besting the runner up cyclist by over 20 minutes. Pro cyclist and pro ironman triathlete – they were clearly competing at another level but I was excited to be racing with both. Heavily favored to win the relay cycling leg, LeMond would be the one to chase, marked by helicopters following him during this nationally televised event.

As it turned out, LeMond's bike had 42 and 53 tooth chainrings and a range of 12 to 24 teeth freewheel gears – a pretty standard road racing setup for the day. I was still stubbornly using a *44* tooth inner chainring, and my 13 to 26 tooth freewheel gears provided some relief at the low end but not much in the middle gears – where I could've used it while climbing. I realized later on that these gears were much better suited to racing in Sacramento – not the *Sierra Nevada!*

Not that it mattered much. As predicted, once the race began *Team Kahlua's* swimmer was one of the first out of the water and Greg LeMond took off, never to be seen much again or caught by anyone, during a race that he later said "was like a long training ride." Clearly in a cycling league of his own, he demonstrated his superiority, dealing with the cold inclement weather and extreme terrain, ultimately riding away from everyone to win the bike leg and set a new course record. Eventual Ironman division winner Scott Molina would also break his own previous record, but finished close to an hour *behind* LeMond on the bike.

Back in the realm of 'thirty-something' amateurs, Noel had put in a remarkable effort, finishing within ten minutes of the lead swimmers. I took our team arm band. "See you in seven hours or so," I said, and rolled away. It was about 8:45 am.

Over my shoulder, I heard him say, "Great – I'll have enough time to go take a nap!"

I considered chasing down world champion professionals – for a moment. Scott Molina had finished the swim in less than an hour, which meant he and Greg LeMond were both already *minutes* up the road. Feeling the adrenaline of the start, I pushed myself but the route out of town included mandatory stops at several intersections. Race officials were enforcing strict disqualification rules – every rider had to come to a complete stop and put a foot down so that course marshals could see a shoe touch the ground.

Every racer lost a bit more time to LeMond as we made it through this 'stop and go' section of the course. Though his eventual winning margin was enough that it made no difference, his bike was the *only* one equipped with the first version of *Look*-style 'clipless' pedals,[14] sparing him this annoyance.

The delays over, I was soon on my way out of South Lake Tahoe and heading up Highway 50 towards Meyers and Highway 89. There I would cross Christmas Valley and begin the steady climb towards the 7,740 ft. Luther Pass. Judging by the helicopters, LeMond was already on the ascent, stringing out some chasers, including not just Scott Molina – but me.

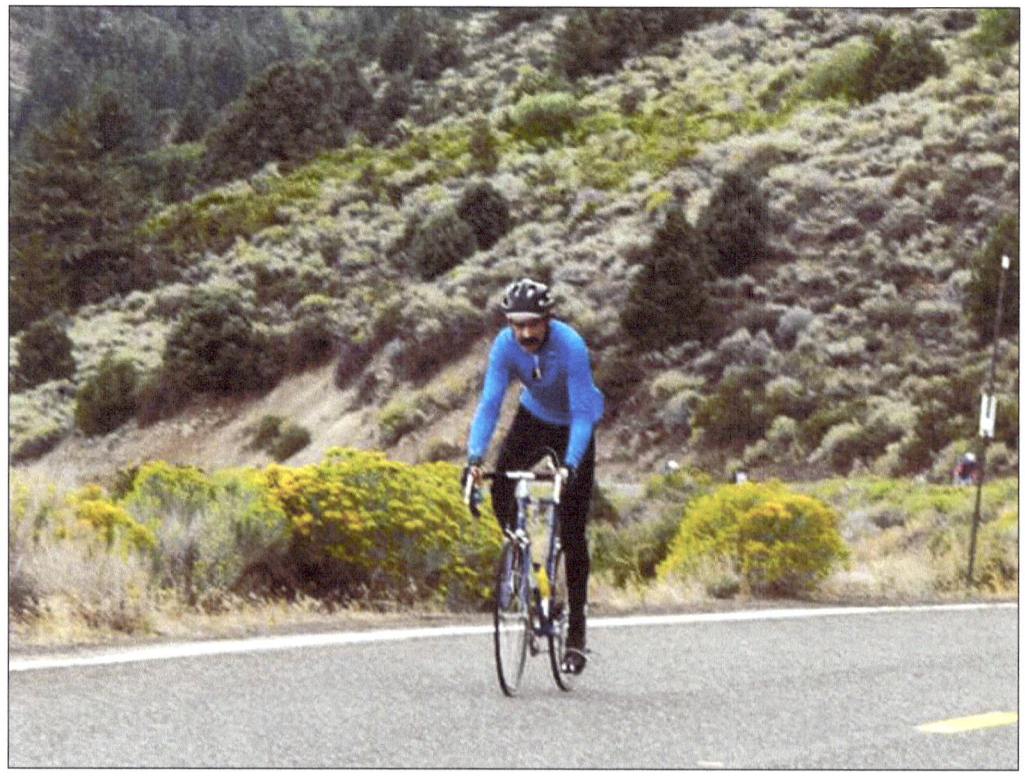

Climbing Luther Pass (Hwy 89).

---

14. *Look* pedals use a spring mechanism and a shoe cleat to allow rapid step-in or twist-out movement's by a rider.

I settled into the 1,500 foot climb and came to my senses about chasing LeMond and Molina on a bike equipped with gears better suited for a flat *criterium* race. There were hours of riding ahead and a 3,300 foot climb over Monitor Pass before climbing Luther Pass a second time from Woodfords – a 2,100 foot climb. My adrenaline leveled off and I went back to my plan of staying in range of the previous top ten finisher's times.

Many of the 1984 elite men and women had finished in six to seven and a half hours. I had decided to keep my time as close to that as I could. With 120 miles, 9,100 feet of climbing, possible inclement weather, mandatory check points at each of the three summits – seven hours seemed good. I wasn't going to catch the top professionals but I was fit, acclimated, and I had trained hard all year. Keeping it around 'lucky seven' was the plan... little did I know what an *unlucky* rendezvous with destiny I would have in almost exactly seven hours.

I still look back on this all day race as one of my best rides ever. The wise old owner at *Dad's Bike Shop* had warned me years earlier, "It's the surprises that getcha," but prior to the triathlon's *surprise* ending for me, every one of those hours had been intense and fantastic – some of my most memorable cycling moments. The first hour included not only the steep climb over Luther Pass but a fast ten mile sinuous descent through Woodfords to Centerville. The landscape was a spectacular palette of yellow, green and brown. Low angled morning sunlight played on the reflective granite. The smell of vaporizing sap on the pine trees wafted over the road. Deer grazed in shaded meadows. The rhythmic sounds of my rolling wheels and breezes moving above were musical. Woodpeckers throttled the trees in the surrounding forest. I felt that state of *'bicycle bliss'* at fifty miles an hour!

As morning progressed, the blue sky filled rapidly with thunder clouds and the main group of racers spent the following two hours getting pelted by rain and hail along the twenty miles of Highway 395, heading south past Double Spring Flat toward Topaz Lake – the race halfway point. At some point, the rain moved through and I began to 'dry out.' I was carrying extra water in my clothing. Strange but true, riding through the day's *first* storm was annoying but the energy felt invigorating and freshened the air. A little over three hours had elapsed.

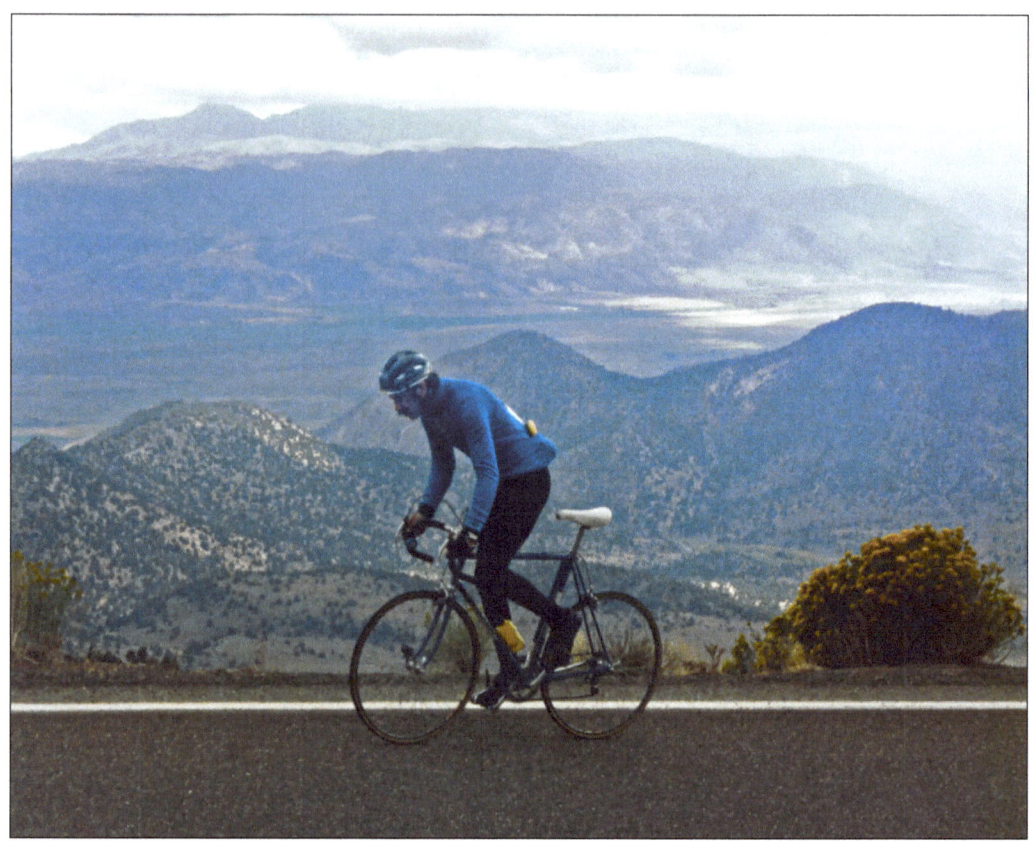

Climbing Monitor Pass (Hwy 89)

The steep 12.5 mile climb over Monitor Pass was a challenge but having just ridden it a few days earlier I knew what to expect. I felt strong and paced myself. The first rain had moved east and created a picturesque backdrop for the climb. The dark clouds and long views towards Nevada from the switchback turns were stunning. After an hour of steady climbing I reached the medical checkpoint just beyond the crest. I was smiling as I came to a halt.

"Your papers, please!" the statuesque young doctor said to me. She laughed and I smiled.

"No – just kidding..." She checked my race number and asked me my name.

"Jon Van Coops," I replied.

"Where are you?" Her assistant was taking my pulse.

"Monitor Pass, Highway 89," My reply was matter-of-fact.

"All is good? Is there anything we can do for you?" she asked.

Smiling awkwardly, I asked, "Is there somewhere I can take a *piss* real quick?"

She paused and then replied in a low voice, "Why don't you just step around the back of my camper here."

When I returned she handed me some folded sheets of newspaper as I was climbing onto my bike. "It's an old motorcycle rider's trick for keeping the chest warm," she said, "You've probably heard about it... I hear it's pretty rainy on the way down to Markleeville."

"Thank you," I replied and tucked several pages of *Tahoe Daily Tribune* under my jersey. Off I went – a little over four hours had now elapsed.

———————

The steep seven mile descent to Markleeville was just as the doctor predicted. The steady pelting with large raindrops and small hailstones made it tough. Tight turns and cattle crossings covered with carpeted sheets of plywood made it impossible to do much more than just roll down the mountain, moving the legs only to corner and maintain balance. Braking in the rain was tricky and my fingers started to cramp. I found myself in a group of racers unable to gain any speed on the downhill.

Fortunately, the rain let up some during the gradual climb west from Markleeville to Turtle Rock Park. With a four mile descent to Woodfords and the steep eight mile climb back to Luther Pass still remaining before the last 18 miles, it seemed certain that my time estimate would be close. The descent from Monitor Pass had slowed the pace for everyone caught in the heavy rain. It was 2 pm – over five hours had now elapsed for me. Racers were soaked!

At his pace of over 25 miles an hour, Greg LeMond had stayed mostly ahead of the rain and already finished the bike race, handing his armband to Team Kahlua's runner *forty five minutes earlier!* LeMond had *smashed* the previous record by over an hour – completing the bike course in 4 hours and 37 minutes! The eventual winner of the Ironman division, Scott Molina, was still out on course, 40 minutes from his arrival at the bike/run transition.

The cold and dark – eight mile 2,100 foot – grinding climb from Woodfords to Luther Pass was followed by the last long descent to Highway 50 at Meyers. The gray skies opened up and I was pelted again by cold rain, turning to light snow on the ten mile downhill. This last push to the Lake took over an hour but my goal was still in range – I'd covered close to 110 miles in six and a half hours. The weather was finally letting up and all that remained before reaching the finish at Stateline was a mostly flat, nine mile section of Pioneer Trail.

———————

Anyone familiar with South Lake Tahoe knows that traffic congestion near the Stateline, Nevada casinos increases on most Saturday afternoons – this one was *no* exception. Main arterial streets typically back up in all directions with vehicles heading to 'the clubs.' Adding the Labor Day holiday and an all day sporting event had amplified the 'stop and go' effect along Highway 50 *and* Pioneer Trail. As I turned onto Pioneer Trail all I could see was a continuous line of sluggish, heavy traffic inching its way along the road. Immediately, I smelled gasoline rich exhaust from auto engines nearly at idle. Waves of heat shimmered above the cars in the distance.

I thought about all I had enjoyed and endured that day – the black and blue skies and fresh mountain air, colors, sounds and smells, rain, hail and snow! The long distance, tough climbs, the grand views... It had been a cold and wet, yet truly 'epic' ride for me. It was easy to ignore the noxious fumes and 'put the hammer down' for the final stretch. I had done what I set out to do. The police directing traffic at Ski Run Boulevard waved me through the intersection. I began hearing the steady cheers of spectators lining the course and loudspeakers booming at Harrah's Casino – the bike race finish – now less than a mile up ahead. It was just after 4 pm.

———————

In the United States, cyclists riding at speed are often keenly aware of parked or stopped cars to their *right*. However, here I was, racing past slow moving cars on my *left,* in a bike lane separated from traffic only by orange plastic cones and a painted white line. After crossing Ski Run Boulevard, I accelerated. The traffic on my immediate left side was literally at a standstill.

Suddenly, the impatient young driver of a Toyota pickup truck attempted to turn right onto to a side street... unfortunately, without looking back *or* signaling. It was the premature end of my race – I was speeding through the same intersection at 25 miles an hour when he crashed into me, sending my bike and me careening to the right and onto the ground.

It was one of a cyclist's worst nightmares! I didn't lose consciousness in the collision but fortunately, I have absolutely *no* memory of the actual impact. The next thing I can recall is looking up from the ground, seeing bright flashes of white light, and asking someone to please loosen the strap on my right pedal so that I could get my foot out of the toe clip. I heard people screaming at the teenage driver of the truck.

"Do you realize what you just did? Man, that dude's been riding all day! What are you doing? There's a race going on here!"

Perhaps luckily for the kid, race monitors began to arrive at the scene to take charge and radioed to police and medical staff, informing them that an accident had occurred.

In the meantime someone helped get my foot loose and I immediately knew I had been seriously injured. I couldn't move my right leg. I realized my upper leg was broken somewhere and all I could do was lie still, holding it as immobile as possible. Soon the police and an ambulance arrived. The EMTs splinted my leg, got me onto a stretcher and before long I was on my way to the nearby Barton Memorial Hospital.

Noel told me later that we did, in fact, have a rendezvous in 'seven hours or so,' just *not* like we had planned... He and his wife had been making their way past the accident scene towards the transition zone at Harrah's Casino when they realized the rider involved was me! By the time that they reached Harrah's the race officials had already notified Shawn that his team's bike rider had been hit by a car.

According to the race rules, our team was 'disqualified' because I didn't complete my leg of the relay and hand off my armband to our team's runner. Technically, since no hand off had occurred Shawn was unable to start the marathon. However, in hindsight now 39 years later, this doesn't really seem fair to any of us. I had ridden over seven hours and all but the very last *half mile* of a 120 mile race. *I was less than two minutes from the finish line!* It would have been much more equitable if Shawn had been allowed to complete the marathon. Then we could have filed a protest regarding the team's disqualification. As it was, none of us had done anything to warrant a 'DQ' but there was nothing we could do about it.

———————

It was such an abrupt and unfortunate turn of events, to say the least. After minutes that seemed like hours, I arrived at the hospital and was quickly seen by Dr. Paul Fry – fortunately for me – a National Laurate orthopedic surgeon from the renowned *Lake Tahoe Fracture Clinic.* Dr. Fry had been one of the medical personnel staffing the mandatory race checkpoints and rushed directly to the hospital when informed that a downed racer was en route.

"I'm pretty sure you fractured your femur," he said, after I described what had happened. "It's going to require surgery... I do several of these procedures a week. Most people can recover well, especially when they're young, like you... Let's go get an x-ray."

On some level, I felt reassured. I was alive – I had no concussion, but I was still in shock and excruciating pain. How could this have happened? I really had no clue about what to expect. I was thirsty and hadn't eaten any real food since early in the morning. My cycling clothes were wet and the room was cold. I couldn't even slide myself onto the x-ray table. Dr. Fry himself, donned a lead vest and 'manhandled' the equipment into a view position from above the gurney. Back in the exam room I waited for him to read the image. The nurses gave me ice chips and cleaned up my minor abrasions.

Dr. Fry was 'hands on' and direct. "Okay, it looks like I thought it would," he said when he returned. "The neck of your femur is broken and there are some fractures in the trochanter area at the top of the hip. This is an image of what it will look like *after* surgery. I did this one last week."

He held up another patient's x-ray, showing what looked like a leg bone with screws and some kind of angled fixture or brace.

"Looks like a serious piece of metal or something," was all I could manage to say.

"Stainless steel," he replied. "Believe me, even ten years ago you would've first had it set and then spent eight months or more somewhere, *in traction*... You'll bounce back from this... Do you want me to do the surgery tonight or tomorrow morning?" His voice conveyed his certainty and my simple choice.

"Do it tonight, please..." My statements were becoming less than ten words long.

As he left the exam room, he gave the nurses instructions, "Okay, give him a shot and get him ready for surgery."

Several nurses went to work right away. One gave me pain meds and got an IV going in my hand. Another asked me about my medical history while a third began cutting off my jersey and cycling clothes with a pair of scissors. The rain and a day's worth of sweat had pretty much soaked my kit. Even my shoes and socks were still wet. She reached the soggy, disintegrating newspaper that I'd tucked under my jersey at Monitor Pass and stopped.

"What's all *this?*" she asked, completely puzzled.

The other two nurses stopped what they were doing and stared curiously at my torso. There were a dozen or more wet pieces of newspaper glued to my chest like papier mâché.

"I guess it's the *Tahoe Daily Tribune*," I halfway chuckled. "It's an old motorcycle rider's trick... to keep the chest warm."

"Looks like it's been under your shirt for a while," she said, and went to work peeling off the shredded pieces of wet newsprint.

The pain meds kicked in and my direct recall of the evening fades quickly from this point. Suffice it to say that several hours later I was waking up in the recovery room after 'successful' surgery. I now had the same hardware in my hip that I'd seen in Dr. Fry's x-ray earlier that evening. I was released following an eight day stay in the hospital and returned home to life on my houseboat in Sausalito.

Of course, *my* story doesn't end there but this story ends because it is about the triathlon and this amazing bike race – a magnificent, memorable ride – and what happened *that* day. The aftermath and recovery from these events, and their influence on my life are topics for separate stories. Looking back, I was fortunate that the crash didn't happen at the *start* of the race. I got to do the entire ride – almost. I learned a ton about friends and family in the ensuing months, and about embracing a healthy dependence on others when you need it. Best of all, I learned about reaching beyond the 'limitations' of injury and continued cycling enthusiastically, even to this day. I always finish telling this story by declaring that "I never rode my bike 200 miles in one day until *after* poppin' the hip."

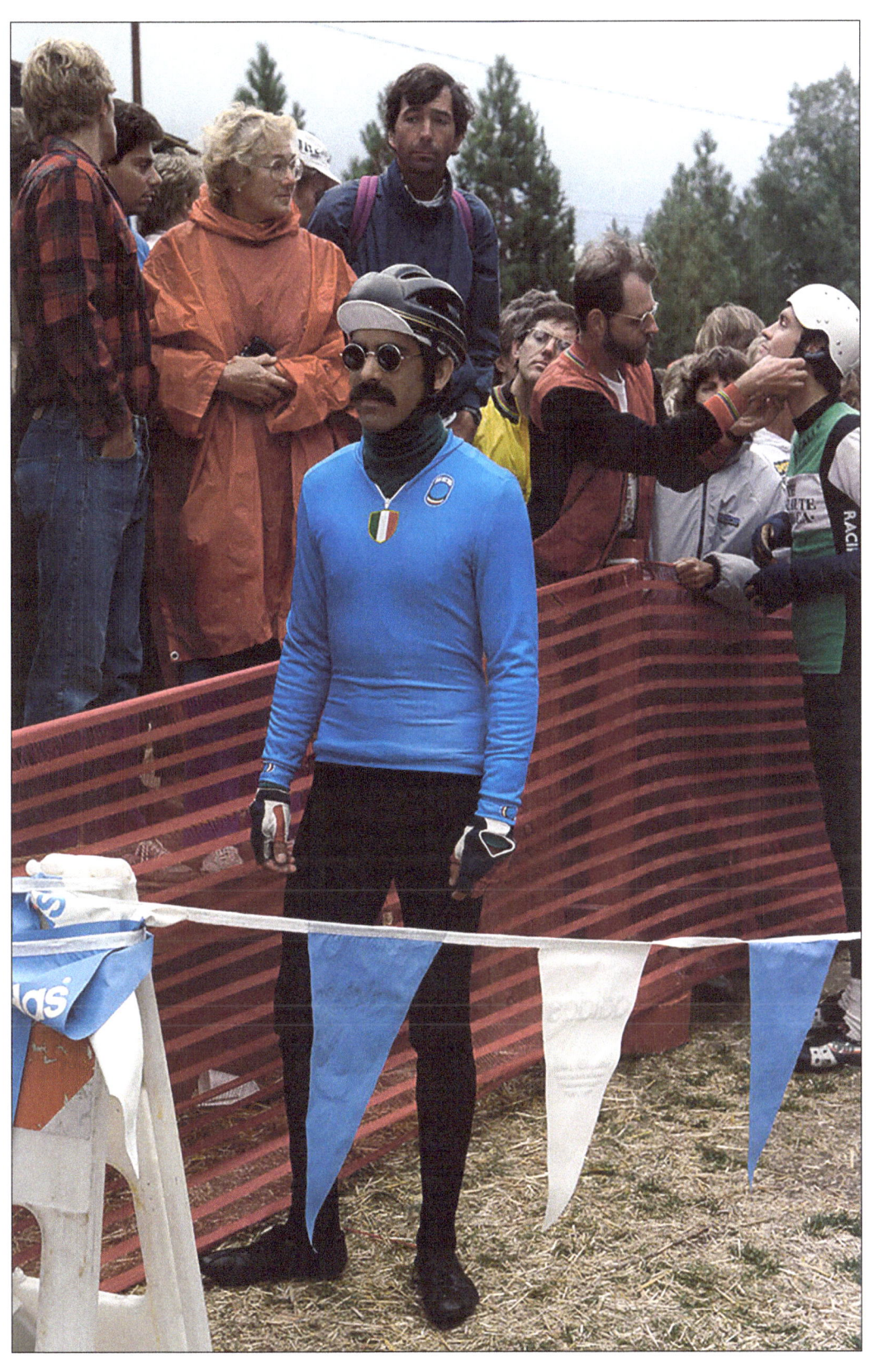

**Awaiting destiny at the *World's Toughest Triathlon*
South Lake Tahoe, Ca, Sept 7, 1985**

Just remember – you can 'git goin' awful fast on a one speed bike

– MARK BEACH, SR.
  Surfboard designer, *Tiki* artist and childhood neighbor

Rolling a Sew-Up (1989)

The year was 1989. It was the era of the 'yuppie' – the *young urban professional.* An employed college graduate, usually under age 35 – upwardly mobile and trying to get there as quickly as possible. Most of my friends and coworkers considered it a serious insult to be called a yuppie, but there was one fellow at work who *wanted* to be a yuppie. He insisted on trying to convince others that they were yuppies, too – and that it was okay. Somehow, he found a list of the ten 'official' characteristics of a yuppie, and proceeded to traverse the office regularly, questioning colleagues in order to determine whether or not they were yuppies. When he came to me, I refused to take the test and told him that there was no way I was a yuppie – by anyone's definition.

"Come on," he said. My coworker was insistent. "You're telling me none of these apply to you? Do you have a *mobile* phone?"

"Of course not," I snapped back.

"Do you own a BMW?" he asked.

"No," I replied sharply. I lived in the very urban city of El Cerrito, owned a small pickup truck and got along just fine taking public transit to work.

"Do you own any property?" he continued down the list.

I had to laugh. "No way," I shot back... I knew he meant a house or land.

"Alright, I guess you're not a yuppie," he said. "Hey, wait a minute – you own bikes, don't you? A lot of bikes, right?"

"Yeah, five bikes – so what?" I said.

"Expensive bikes, right? Like *thousand dollar* bikes?" He kept probing.

"Okaaay?" I said, drawing it out like a question... but I knew he had me.

"You're a *bike* yuppie!" he almost yelled it, grinning ear to ear and proclaiming, "Hey everybody! Jon's a *bike* yuppie! I knew it!"

"Get outa' here!" I growled at him, "Yuppies make over *fifty* thousand a year!"

Nevertheless he was correct. I *had* assembled a small collection of fine, expensive bikes: my new *Colnago* racing bike, a striking red 1979 *Masi Gran Criterium,* a midnight blue 1979 *Santana Marathon* tandem, my extremely rare and beautiful 1939 *Schwinn Century* balloon tired cruiser and most recently – an undeniable prize – my sharp looking dark green 1979 *Schwinn Paramount* track racing bike, complete with track wheels, *'sew-up'* tires, and a single fixed gear. I could afford to indulge myself in bicycles and I was doing it – without any hesitation. The *Paramount* was my latest 'project' bike. A bike yuppie – indeed I was. I had decided to buy this one speed bike for flatland training out on the road. But it had no brakes – and I bought it anyway.

Track racing bicycles are not equipped with brakes, so frames built for the track typically have no brake caliper mounts for either wheel. In the case of the *Paramount,* however, I would soon find how lucky I was that the fork crown had been drilled out to accept a front brake caliper. Hindsight also makes it clear that I was fortunate in having the sense or premonition that, should I add one, it would later come in handy.

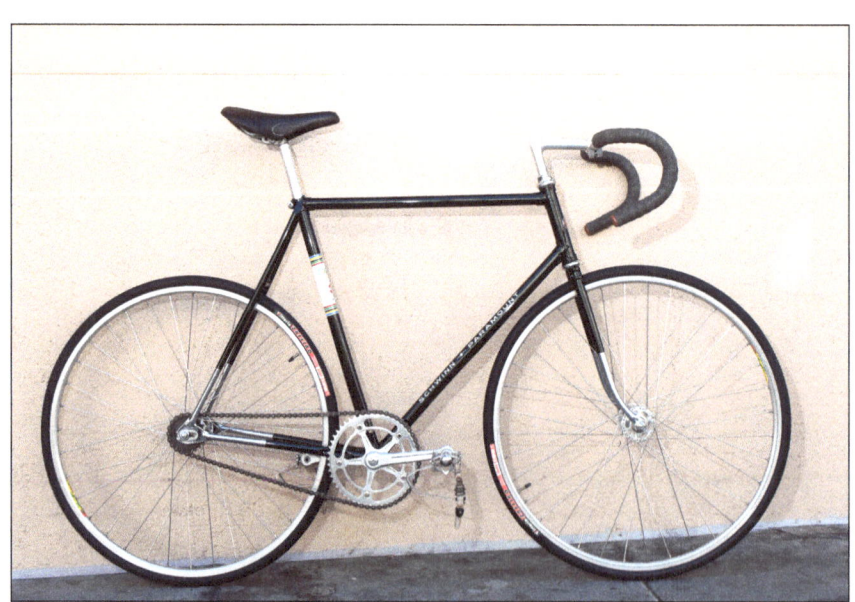

1979 *Schwinn Paramount* track racing bike

I immediately installed an old *Campagnolo* front brake and lever that I had lying around, which emboldened me to take my first *fixed gear* bike ride out on the street. But it would be during that very first ride on this beautiful machine that I would unexplainably avoid a bizarre and potentially disastrous downhill crash, while simultaneously learning some important lessons about tubular tires and wheels – sew-ups, that is.

Anyone who's ridden a bike equipped with sew-up tires is likely to know that not only is the tube sewn inside the tire casing and tread but the tire itself is mounted by gluing it to the wheel rim. Of course, a more standard wheel has a separate tube and a tire with a circular wire bead on both sides which holds it to the inside of the rim. A dedicated cyclist could likely have a long discussion about the relative merits and characteristics of riding on sew-ups versus the usual 'clincher' tires but the two major points for this story are that track bikes of the day used sew-ups almost exclusively, and that mounting a sew-up tire requires the use of a special liquid glue, ironically called 'rim cement.'

Rim cement – it was my downfall from the beginning. Red, 'gooey' and flowing when it's fresh out of the tube – noxious fumes. Once it's begun to dry, it is impossible to get off hands or pants or bike parts without solvent. Nasty, sticky stuff – difficult to work with. Nevertheless, there I was on a Thursday night gluing on a brand new pair of fifty dollar tubular tires so I could try out my *new* track bike on the road that Saturday morning.

I had been riding indoors on my 'rollers' for the first two weeks after buying it – riding the fixed gear setup felt as if you were really connected to the bike. I already felt comfortable pedaling for a half an hour during my stationary workouts. I could carefully ride 'no hands' and was anxious to try my new bike out on the street.

Saturday arrived and everything was a go – or so I thought. Somehow, it hadn't occurred to me that it might be a good idea to let rim cement dry for more than just 24 hours before using the wheels. I knew enough about sew-ups to first mount new tires *without* glue to stretch them for a couple of days before cementing but the importance of glue 'drying time' had escaped me. In the morning air the new tires felt solidly stuck – I pumped the tires to 110 pounds of air pressure and took off.

What an incredible ride! Immediately, I was 'at one' with the bike – locked in to a fixed gear. I was feeling the road throughout my body. It was the same feeling I'd noticed riding the rollers but amplified. I was pedaling the bike and feeling propelled forward by the bike's momentum at the same time. It felt *really* good. The bike was super lightweight and responsive to my every move. The mid range gearing and shorter crank arms made it easy to accelerate. The streets seemed as if they were my personal racing track. I had to keep myself from ignoring stop signs and traffic lights – after all – I had a front brake only.

Half an hour later I was unconsciously drifting away from the flatlands and traffic of west Berkeley and headed up Tunnel Road, a quiet, less traveled route my friend Tom and I often used when we were riding to Grizzly Peak Boulevard, at the crest of the Berkeley hills. Soon I was halfway up the hill, sweating and having to stand up and pedal on the steepest sections, but I was loving it. The bike performed well and was so light and responsive and quiet – all I could hear was the sound of the tires contacting the pavement, resonating through the entire bike creating a sound like a rhythmic low throaty bellows, the perfect background to the buzzing insects and birds calling in the surrounding trees and brush. I felt winded but satisfied as I reached the intersection with Grizzly Peak Boulevard and turned north along a flatter section heading towards Tilden Regional Park.

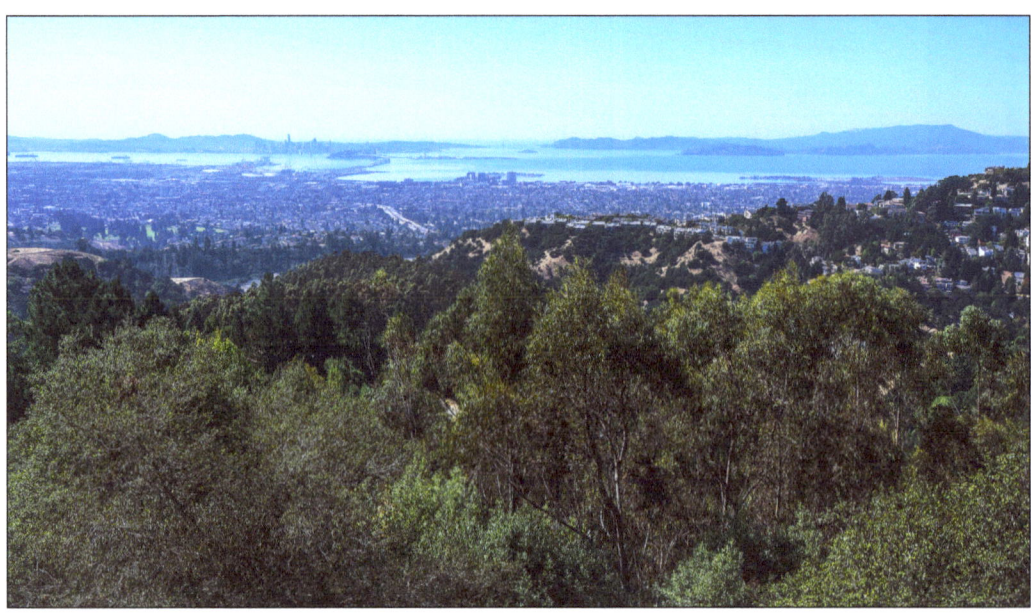

View from the Berkeley Hills towards the Bay, San Francisco and Marin County

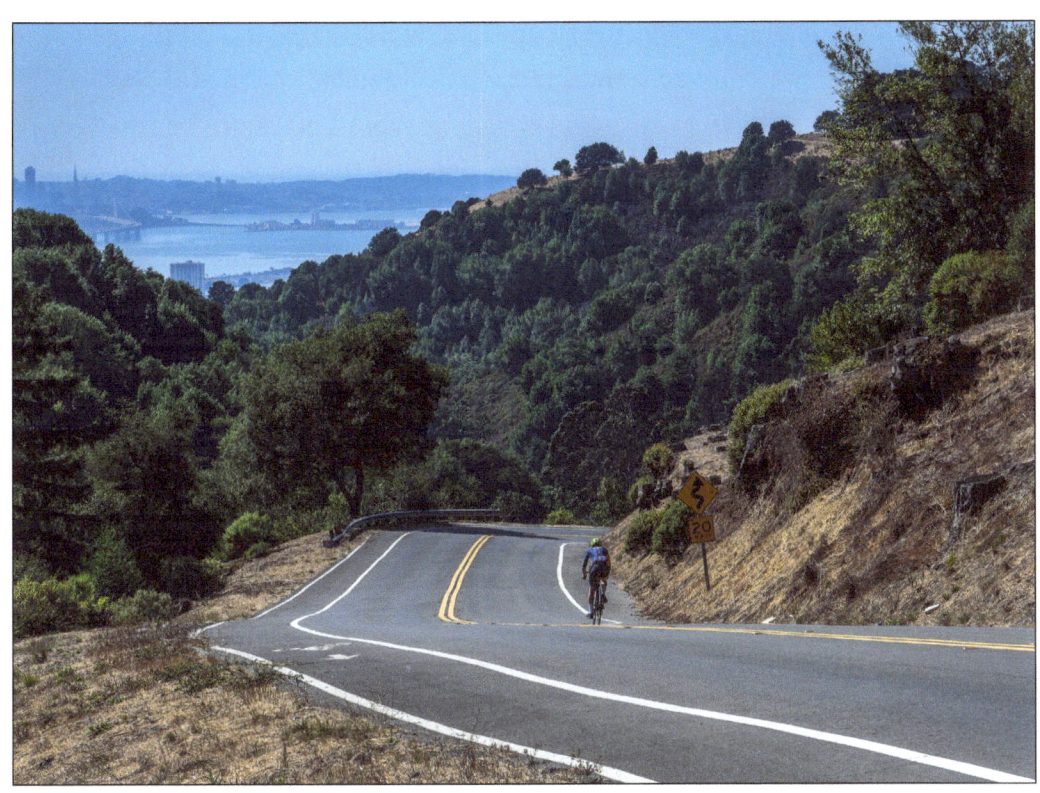

Claremont Canyon Road, Berkeley, Ca

It suddenly occurred to me that I would now have to *descend* a thousand feet or so to Berkeley to get back home, no matter which way I went. *Oops!* I realized that, on this fixed gear bike, it meant that I would be rolling downhill as slowly as possible, applying as much back pressure to the pedals as I had the knee strength for and simultaneously using the front brake to further keep my speed low. I approached the left turn to Claremont Canyon Road which would take me steeply down behind the Claremont Hotel to the relative safety of Berkeley's flatlands. Thinking that I preferred to get it over with sooner rather than later, I turned left and realized right away that I was in for a *real* adventure.

What happened next quickly became a *surreal* experience with a very real lesson in how *not* to ride downhill on a track bike – or any bike – with freshly glued sew-ups. Descending along the steep top section of Claremont Canyon Road made it immediately clear that I was not going to be able to control my speed by applying back pressure on the pedals. The wheels were actually turning my legs and the more back pressure I applied, the more I was forced up, off the saddle. All I could do was brake hard and pedal as slowly as possible.

Descending through the steep, tight turns I realized something was terribly wrong with my front wheel. I looked down and saw that the tire was in the process of rolling over in place on the rim. The sidewall and underside of the tire was in contact with the ground. The tire tread had rotated sideways and was hitting the blade of the fork. Sticky glue was smeared on the sidewall which began picking up road debris. It was obvious that the hard steady braking had heated up the rim enough to melt the rim cement. The tire was no longer held in place and fortunately, the 110 lbs. of air pressure in the tire had somehow kept it on the rim.

There was no other choice but to try to stop the bike, and fast! Any other maneuver was to invite an absolute disaster of a crash. The first thing I had to do was loosen my toe clip straps so I could get my feet out of the toe clips. Imagine riding down a steep hill on a fixed gear bike, braking with the left hand and trying to loosen *both* toe clip straps! I could only reach my shoes at the top of a pedal stroke, so it took several revolutions to get them loosened. It was an amazing feat in hindsight – one I seriously doubt could be repeated.

Next was getting my shoes out of the toe clips and me off the bike. The incline lessened and I took the opportunity to slow as much as I could. Then, in a matter of seconds I unclipped from the pedals and dismounted in a bizarre jump, letting my bike fall. There I stood, amazed and unhurt, staring at my bicycle.

The road was steep and there were leaves and thick debris on the roadside from the surrounding Eucalyptus trees. It was the era of stiff nylon-soled bike shoes and as I took a step towards my bike, I slipped like someone had 'pulled the rug' from under me and landed square on my backside. I wasn't hurt and laughed out loud. I was pissed and felt stupid but simultaneously grateful for having not been injured.

Embarrassed but luckily without an audience, I got up and walked in short sidesteps to where my bike had made a soft landing. The front tire was still completely inflated but had rolled around onto the sidewall almost everywhere except at the valve stem. There was glue on the brake pads and caliper arms. I knew I would be there for a while. I began to pick rocks and debris off the inner side of the tire and carefully repositioned the tire so that the tread would roll – not the sidewall. Glue was everywhere and an old cotton handkerchief became my best friend as I used it to wipe glue off the brake arms and tires.

Finally, everything was ready for my attempt at riding the rest of the way down Claremont Canyon Road. My hands were sticky, there was glue on the tread of the front tire but there was nothing left to delay me further. I made sure not to gain any speed, essentially crawling along the rest of the descent to Ashby Avenue. I had to remain careful, watching the position of the front tire on the rim, using the brake as little as possible and not allowing the momentum from the incline to force me to pedal at a higher cadence. It was slow and excruciating to both balance and move forward foot by foot. Eucalyptus pods appeared on the shady, wet section of road above the Claremont Hotel. It was tense and difficult – and then it was over.

Well, not exactly... I reached Ashby Avenue and stopped to let my hands and arms take a rest from their flexed positions. I looked at the front tire. It had started to rotate again on the lower section of the descent. Taking off my gloves, I spent the next five minutes or so repositioning the tread section of the tire to face outward again, an exercise that I would soon repeat, and repeat again, a total of *eight* times before I got home to El Cerrito!

Later as I cleaned the sticky mess of rim cement from my hands and bicycle, I reflected.

"What is the lesson here? – what do I learn from *this* one?" The 'sew-ups and glue' lesson was obvious and so was the one about hill climbing on a fixed gear bike. It could have been a serious, ugly crash, yet I had not been injured at all. Then suddenly – I got it. I was fortunate enough to be there in my garage contemplating a *bonafide* bike yuppie's solution: Get a new set of wheels with 'clincher' rims so it can't happen again... I made my purchase *right away.*

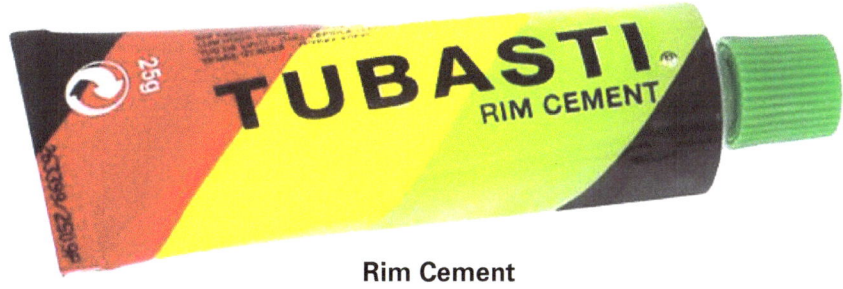

Rim Cement

*What really counts is not how often
you were on the ground but how many times
you got up and kept rolling*

– JVC

Hookin' Handlebars (1990)

It was during the Spring of 1990 that I decided it had been long enough since I'd ridden my bike seriously in the Sierra Nevada, California's eastern high mountains. My almost annual ritual of cycling vacations near Lake Tahoe had temporarily ended with my hip fracture there racing in a triathlon during late 1985. Now five years had gone by and I was ready to attempt riding the 'three pass' version of the *Markleeville Death Ride,* known alternatively as the *'Tour of the California Alps'* – the famous day long event – climbing to the major highway passes that traverse the region south of the lake.[15] The original hardware in my hip had been successfully removed in 1989 and I was riding my repainted and upgraded 1979 *Masi Gran Criterium* every chance I could. It was time to get back to the mountains.

What a beautiful and comfortable bicycle this *Masi* was! Just as with my old *Peugeot,* I rode this bike many hundreds of happy miles and eventually loaned it – long term – to a friend who did likewise. The back story about the *Masi* begins with the aftermath of that same 1985 triathlon accident. As I recovered from the crash and subsequent hip surgery I steadily progressed enough to begin riding a stationary bike and purchased an early version of a direct drive indoor trainer called The Road Machine. My *Colnago Superissimo* racing frame was being repainted and I was impatient to get a bike on the trainer and try it but *I needed a bike!*

Back in the day there were many, many 'Bike for Sale' ads in the various cycling newspapers and racing publications. I scoured the ads and soon hit the jackpot: A 1979 *Masi Gran Criterium* for $300! "What the *hell?* – why isn't it more?" I thought. I knew the frame alone was worth that. If it also had racing wheels and components it was worth twice that much. I *had* to look into it.

The Mill Valley doctor who answered the phone told me that he'd originally purchased two *Gran Criteriums* – one for himself and the other for his wife. Both were metallic blue and equipped with the best *Campagnolo Record* components of the

---

15. Monitor Pass, Ebetts Pass and Carson Pass.

day. He was selling his after denting the top tube in a slow speed collision with his open garage door while the bike, without its front wheel, was mounted on his car's roof rack! I pictured the event as he described it. *Ouch!* He assured me the frame had not been broken but he had already purchased a new bike and was getting 'encouragement' from his wife to sell this one.

I was more than intrigued – a 60 cm frame was slightly larger than my *Colnago* but the parts alone were clearly worth his asking price. I arranged to see it right away. The dent turned out to be a noticeable triangle shaped flat spot – about the size of a quarter – located roughly a third of the distance behind the handlebars on the top tube. It was obvious to the eye but the tube itself looked straight and the paint at both the head tube and seat tube lugs looked solid and uncracked. The doctor and I were about the same height and I stood over the top tube in my street shoes before deciding that I could easily manage the slightly larger frame size.

I had brought along $300 in cash expecting to use it all and I offered him $250, thinking he would want a bit more. To my surprise, he didn't. Instead, his response was "Sure, that's close enough. Thank God I'll get the space back in my garage." I felt a bit awkward as I handed him thirteen $20 bills but he quickly dug a ten out of his pocket. I thanked him and was soon on my way home, already planning my move – frame repair and a paint job.

I rode the *Masi* on my new turbo trainer just several weeks before contacting my long time acquaintance and legendary East Bay frame builder Bernie Mikkelsen. It might have been mostly cosmetic damage but I wanted the frame's top tube replaced and I arranged to meet him at his Alameda shop. His eyes lit up some when he saw the bike and he proceeded to tell me that this same *Masi* was used in the much loved cycling film *Breaking Away*, in which the kid playing the main part wins the big race riding an identical model *Gran Criterium*. Then, in a familiar Bernie fashion, he put my feet right back on the ground when he showed me his "Box of Shame," literally a wooden wine box full of broken frame parts, lugs, bottom brackets, fork crowns, all from 'high end' frames that failed and ended up as his repair jobs.

I looked through the pieces with the most expensive Italian names, including *Masi*. I could see the gaps in the brazing and other flaws that likely led to their failure. My romantic attachment to Italian made bicycle frames shifted abruptly. Bernie noticed my expression as he leaned over and checked the serial number stamped into the bottom bracket of my 'Italian stallion.' "Don't worry," I remember him saying, "This one was made in here in southern California... might have better brazing than some of the older ones."

Two weeks later I had the fork and frame with new top tube ready for painting. Rick Stefani from *D&D Cycles* in San Lorenzo, California was my next call, having done his superb work repainting my *Colnago Superissimo* after being recommended by Bernie Mikkelsen and Tony Tom, owner of *A Bicycle Odyssey*, in Sausalito. I had decided that I wanted the *Masi* painted red and Rick absolutely outdid himself. He used multiple coats of *Imron* paint that gave an irridescent quality to its finish, with bright yellow decals and paint details at the lugs, bottom bracket cutout and frame flourishes. The decals were perfectly placed. The clean lines and tight frame geometry, fat seat stays and raked fork really stood out in red. The clear finish was so strong that I rode this bike for years without scratching or chipping the paint.

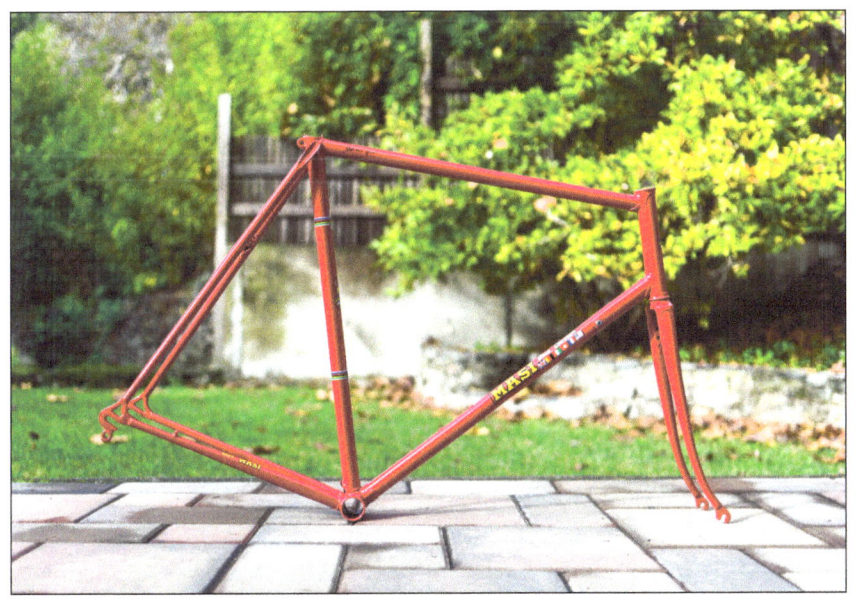

1979 *Masi Gran Criterium* frameset
(painted by Rick Stefani – D & D Cycles)

The story returns to the Spring of 1990 with me living in the East Bay, riding my *Masi* and training for the *Markleeville Death Ride.* Having sold my *Colnago Superissimo* to a student colleague at work several years earlier I was no longer pushing such tough gears up the hills. Instead, the *Masi's* 40 tooth inner chainring provided me with perfect gearing for my climbs through Berkeley and beyond. Since it had become my steady road bike I made a few component upgrades – swapping in a *Campagnolo Super Record* rear derailleur, Cinelli stem and 'aero' brake levers fitted to *Modolo* handlebars. Visually stunning, this bike was an absolute beauty in red and yellow. It shifted and handled like the racing bike it was.

So there I was, one warm and sunny Saturday morning with my longtime friend Shawn Ridley, heading out from his place in Hercules on my *Masi* to do a ride known as 'Morgan Territory.' It's a long, tough loop that encircles and climbs over the eastern shoulder of Mount Diablo in eastern Contra Costa County – requiring about five hours for most riders. We were strong and fit, like 'thirty-something' sporting titans and agreed that the course would be great training for the *Markleeville Death Ride.* However, as destiny would have it, we had just started our ride when we both hit the deck hard – with no one to blame but ourselves.

It's one of those things you learn quickly when riding in groups or with others... If the lead rider sees that it's clear to roll through a stop sign or yellow traffic signal light at an intersection and continues riding, then the other riders continue as well. There's a sort of 'safety in numbers' element to it but there's also a decision made by anyone right behind or alongside the front rider to follow the leader. However, on this particular day, at this particular intersection, it didn't work out that way.

We had been pacing each other out of town on a straight flat stretch of Pinole Valley Road – rolling at nearly twenty miles an hour. Shawn accelerated, overtaking me on the left as we approached a broad intersection. Just as he began crossing, the traffic light turned from green to yellow. I took it as an indication of his decision to continue and instinctively went with him. Suddenly he changed his mind, slowed and veered right, instantly hooking his handlebars on my brake levers and pulling us both to the ground in a great tumble.

The crash happened quickly – but felt like slow motion. It must have looked spectacular to the front row of auto drivers waiting at the intersection. Two cyclists – apparently training – crash into *each other* in the middle of an intersection and crumple to the pavement – with no cars involved! Water bottles rolling in random directions! My adrenaline rush was accompanied by feelings of stupidity and embarrassment as we disentangled the bikes. It was all over in a moment but seemed to take us minutes to get out of the street.

I had toppled onto Shawn, which meant I got the bumps and he got the scrapes – left knee and elbow. He also had scraped some paint but the bikes were otherwise fine. My bumps would turn to bruises but I was otherwise unscathed and I rotated my handlebars back to their proper position. Shawn straightened his brake levers and wiped off silver dollar-size abrasions. Without much discussion or hesitation, we decided to continue the ride.

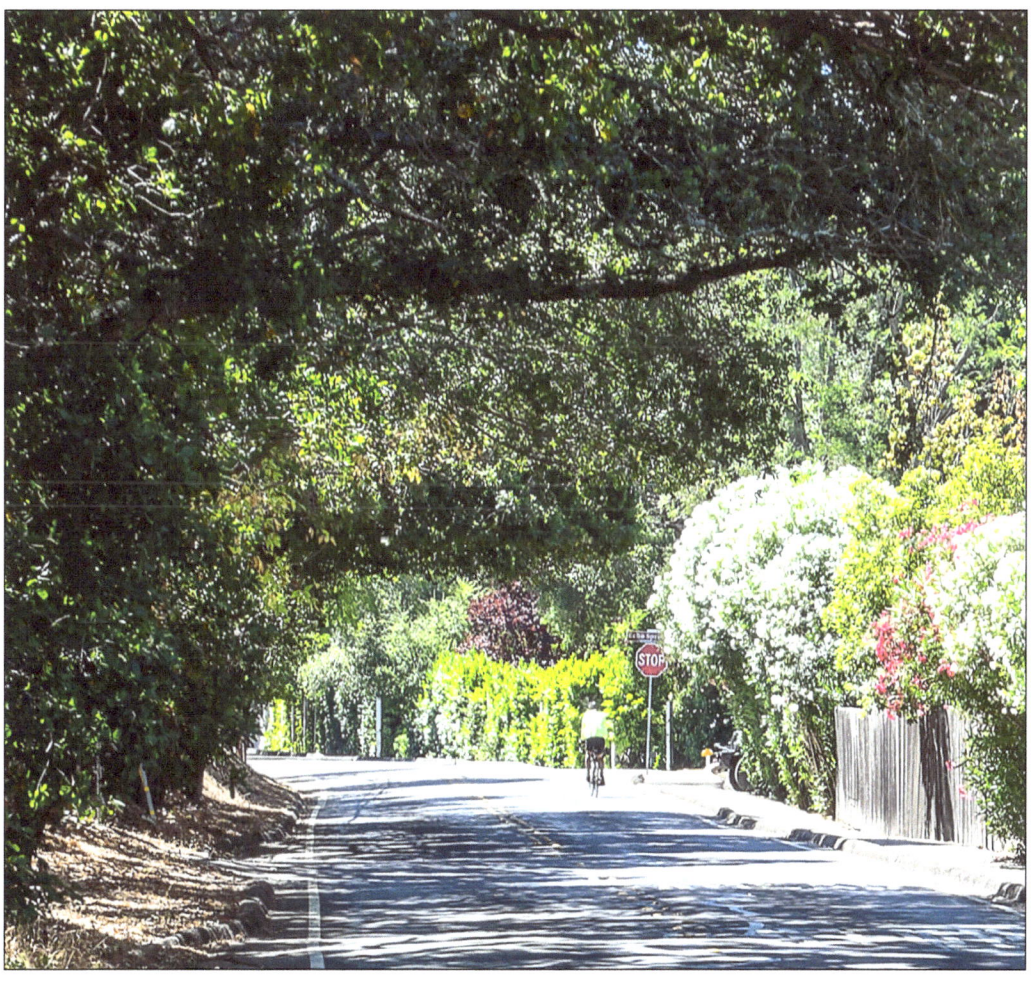

Reliez Valley Road, Contra Costa County

We made our way uneventfully through the Alhambra and Reliez Valleys, then on through Pleasant Hill and Concord. I could feel the temperature rising steadily as we reached the town of Clayton. Surely, the climb up and over Morgan Territory Road would be a hot one. Fortunately, I had two tall water bottles along with my usual applesauce and water concoction in a third – I would need *all* of them.

The next section of the ride was a cruise southeasterly through horse ranches and small farms followed by a climb, first gradual and then steep, into what is now the Morgan Territory Regional Preserve. We took a rest at the equestrian staging area, the highest elevation and halfway point of our ride.

After a stretch, some water and half a banana, it was time to check the tires and begin the return leg of the ride. Shawn was looking pretty red in the face and I knew it was still a long way back – with likely heat and headwinds. We topped off the water bottles and continued south on Morgan Territory Road beginning the long descent to the outskirts of Livermore. The speed felt great and though I was starting to feel some soreness in the bruised places, the fast downhill to Manning Road was 'payback' for all the climbing we had done. We turned right at the base of the hill and began the trek west into a steady headwind.

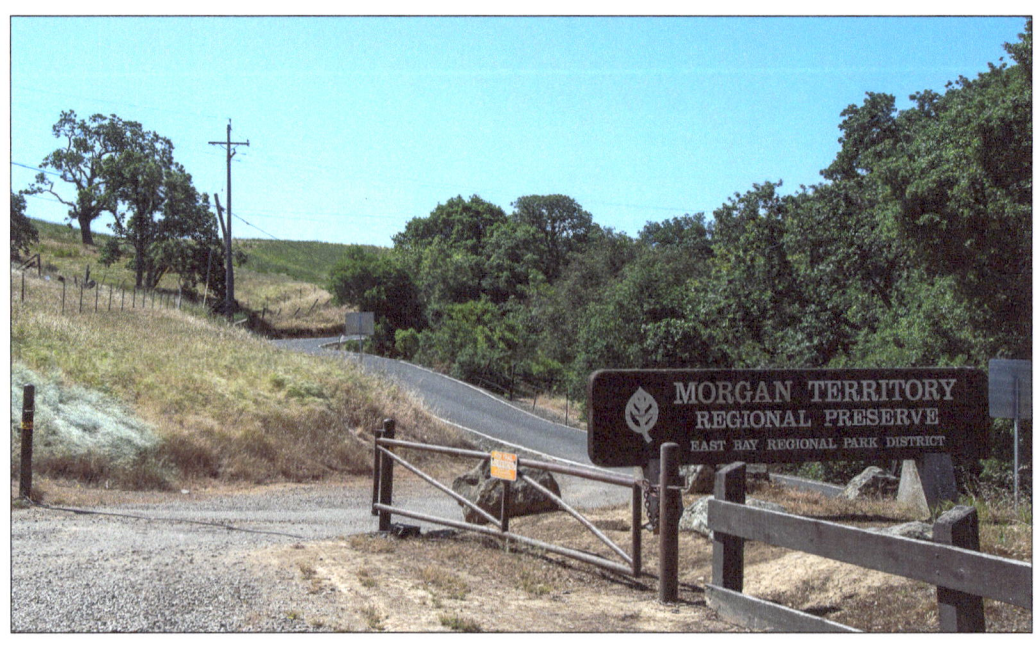

Morgan Territory Regional Preserve, east Contra Costa County

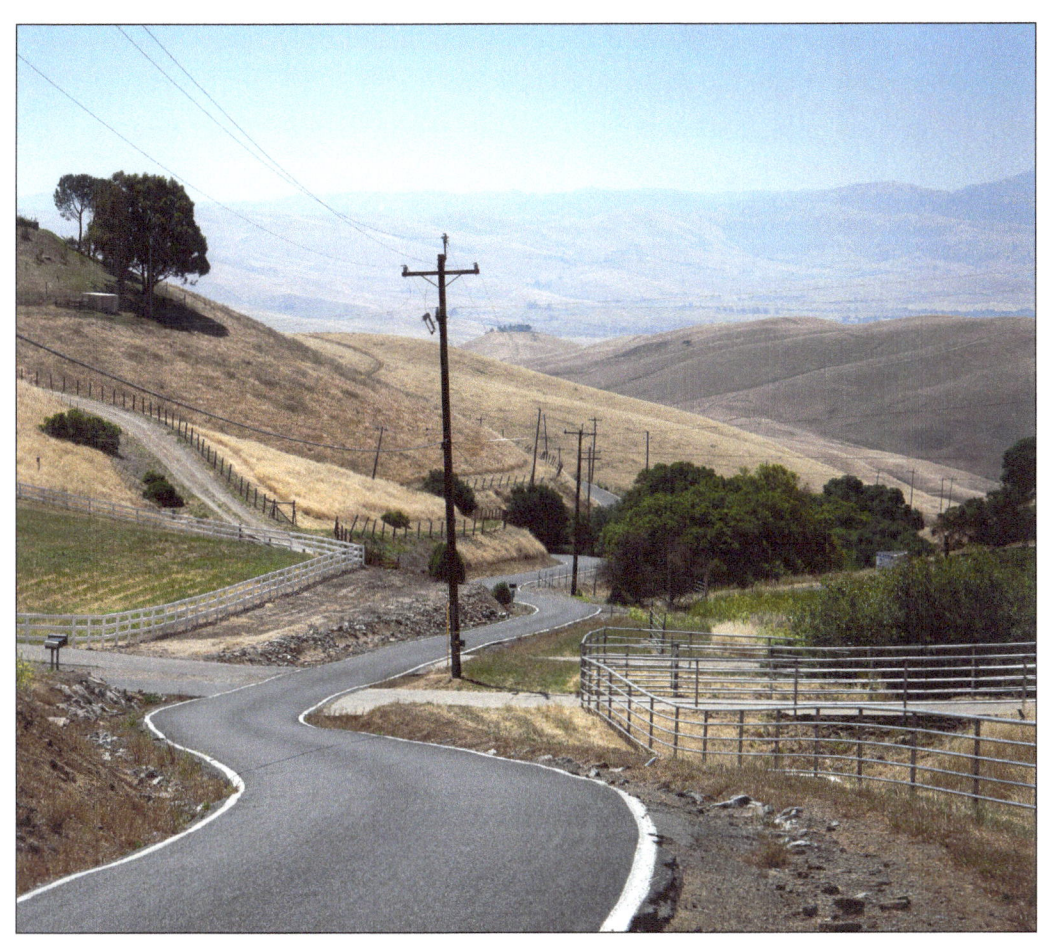
Morgan Territory Road, east Contra Costa County

The highlight of the ride for me happened next. A gap was opening between Shawn and me as we punched into the wind along Camino Tassajara and I decided to slow a bit so he could catch me. A single rider approaching 'flew' by us heading in the opposite direction. I saw that he was on a blue *Colnago* and somehow I realized that I'd just serendipitously crossed paths with *my old bike*! Without hesitating, I yelled out my former student's last name and sure enough – he stopped and turned around.

It was a great to have a short visit with Dave Zender and exciting to hear that he was putting in some good miles on the *Colnago*. The bike fit him well and he was enjoying the *Superissimo* as much as I had. He was slightly shorter than I am but solid and strong enough to push that tough 44 tooth inner chainring up the hills. After five minutes or so chatting in the wind I could see Shawn was splashing water on his face and neck. We said our 'bonne route' to Dave and pushed on towards Blackhawk and Alamo.

Heat, headwinds and climbing were the only fare on the afternoon menu as we meandered north through Walnut Creek and Lafayette. The winding descent along Happy Valley Road into Briones Regional Park that followed was not so 'happy' either – the pavement was rough and broken. Four hours in the saddle had both of us approaching our limits.

After the final climb over Lawson Hill we were 'officially' done – *spent*. The heat and effects of the minor crash had been with us all day and now extracted their full toll. Shawn ran out of water and hit his 'red line' with less than 10 miles left to ride. At Alhambra Valley Road his legs cramped badly. I left him lying in a shady spot alongside the road with my last half-full water bottle and rode on. My legs felt like cement but I was on a mission to get to a pay phone so I could call my buddy's wife and ask if she would pick us up. I arrived at the outskirts of Pinole, made my call and Sydney answered.

Another ten minutes passed and she arrived at the gas station where I sat waiting in the shade of the phone booth. I got my bike into the van quickly and climbed into the back seat. My jersey was streaked with salty, dried sweat. I told her where I had left Shawn and we were there in five minutes. As we rounded the last turn I saw Shawn up off the ground, stretching and looking his bike over. After a difficult ride like this and our early mishap, I couldn't help but feel some sense of accomplishment – despite the chopped ending.

Back at their house the three of us couldn't help but reflect a bit on the ride. Shawn remarked that despite the early tumble, the last half was what had completely "kicked his ass." Sydney – also a competitive athlete – couldn't help but remind us that we had both been dehydrated and were really lucky that she was home when I called. My take was that the cycling gods could be cruel. The message was clear – titans fall too – sooner or later. It was another one of those days with a lesson: *What really counts is not how often you were on the ground but how many times you got up and kept rolling.*

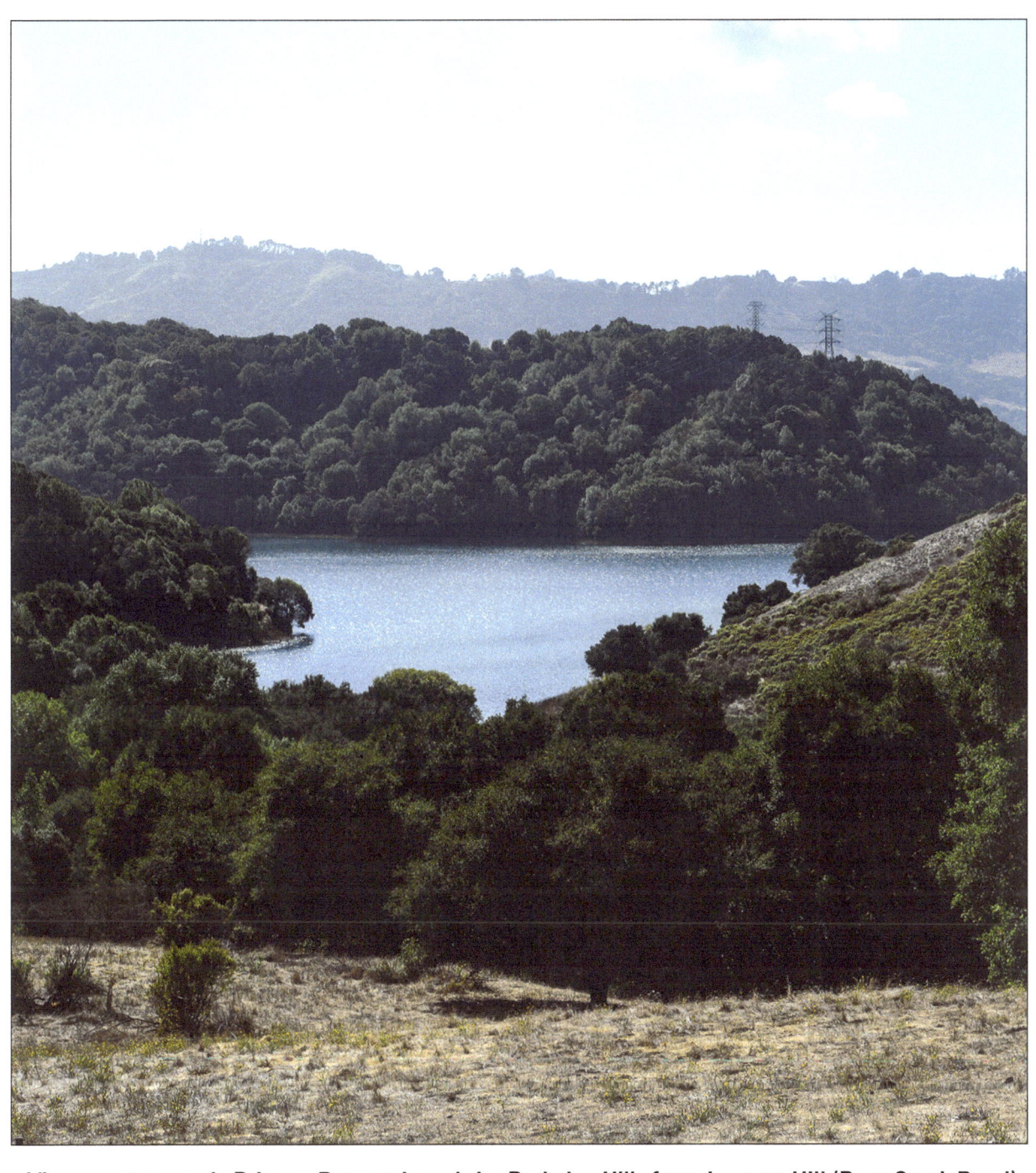
View west towards Briones Reservoir and the Berkeley Hills from Lawson Hill (Bear Creek Road)

Quake or shake, sunny or rainy, we have to flow with time for the next smile

– *Critical Mass* participants
　In Kathmandu, Nepal

Critical Mass (1992)

In the United States, bicycle racing experienced more of a 'boom' than a 'blossoming' during the 1980s. The USA hosted the summer 1984 games of the XXIII Olympiad in Los Angeles where USA cyclists won gold and silver medals in both road and track events. In 1983, Greg LeMond became the first ever USA winner of the men's professional road race at the World Cycling Championships and three years later, won the fabled *Tour de France*. It was the dawn of triathlon and the heyday of the *Coors Classic* stage race from California to Colorado. The 1987 World Cycling Championships were held in Colorado. New regional races also emerged in the Midwest and on the East Coast, adding to a list of venerable local races in the USA that had somehow survived in relative obscurity during the several preceding decades. Bike racing was in the spotlight and flourishing.

It wasn't just bike *racing* that boomed. Cycling as a sportive activity for adults surged. The entire industry experienced a period of growth. Many people in the United States were awakening to cycling as a healthy way to spend leisure time and – for an increasing number of urban workers – a way to commute. Unlike the 1960s when riding a bike to work was viewed as quirky, employers now encouraged the practice – some providing bike parking and other amenities. Even the State of California had issued 'English Racer' style three speed bicycles with baskets and bungee cords to many of its departments and agencies. Helmet wearing civil servants used them regularly in Sacramento, San Francisco and other cities as an alternative to driving cars for local work related travel.

By 1992, I had been riding the San Francisco Bay Area's roads for over 20 years. It was clear to me by then that cycling in the City and other urban centers had become more challenging than ever. San Francisco bicyclists, including myself, found themselves having 'close calls' or collisions on streets that were never designed to accommodate bicyclists. A year earlier I had moved from Marin to the hilly, gridded streets and densely populated neighborhood of Nob Hill. I could now attest to the many risks of riding in the City.

Even with the growing number of signed bike lanes, riding in many parts of the City remained unsafe when it should have become more convenient. Along with the usual obstacles,[16] urban cyclists faced constant hazards maneuvering around double parked delivery trucks and articulated buses, inattentive drivers opening doors or turning suddenly without a signal or indication. Commuting by bicycle was a tense, high alert type of riding. Fortunately, I could routinely walk downtown to work and rode only on occasion. Helmets and other safety gear had become common by the early 1990s but overall, city cyclists seemed more vulnerable. Paradoxically, the significantly greater numbers of cyclists had *not* produced more legitimacy for bicycles as two wheeled vehicles with 'rights to the road.' Something had to give!

———————

Critical Mass began in San Francisco, California on September 25, 1992. It first evolved from an experiment known as *'Commute Clot,'* a decentralized direct action event held that last Friday of September during the evening commute. Initially just a few dozen cyclists were involved. The goal was to effect changes in the way that vehicle traffic and circulation were being managed throughout the City. "We're not blocking traffic, we *ARE* traffic!" was one of the early responses to the criticisms of motorists and authorities. *Commute Clot* doubled its size in October. The fact that it took place a day before Halloween brought a celebratory element to the event. Most of the riders wore costumes. I found out about it and couldn't resist – a friend and I rode my tandem dressed up as Dracula and a cowl-hatted witch.

The *Commute Clot* became *Critical Mass* and a regular event for me. The first rides had all the magic and excitement one might imagine and something else. Each was a serious protest and a mass bike ride but also created an energized, public *moving* space, where people and bicycles became rolling art. The atmosphere felt spontaneous and unpredictable. There was openness and freedom – amazing things happened. There were dozens of creatively masterful and strange looking custom bicycles and people! Every month I witnessed something different. I looked forward to riding in *Critical Mass* and printed flyers about future rides.

---

16. Debris, damaged pavement, steel grates, railroad tracks, utility infrastructure (manhole covers), etc.

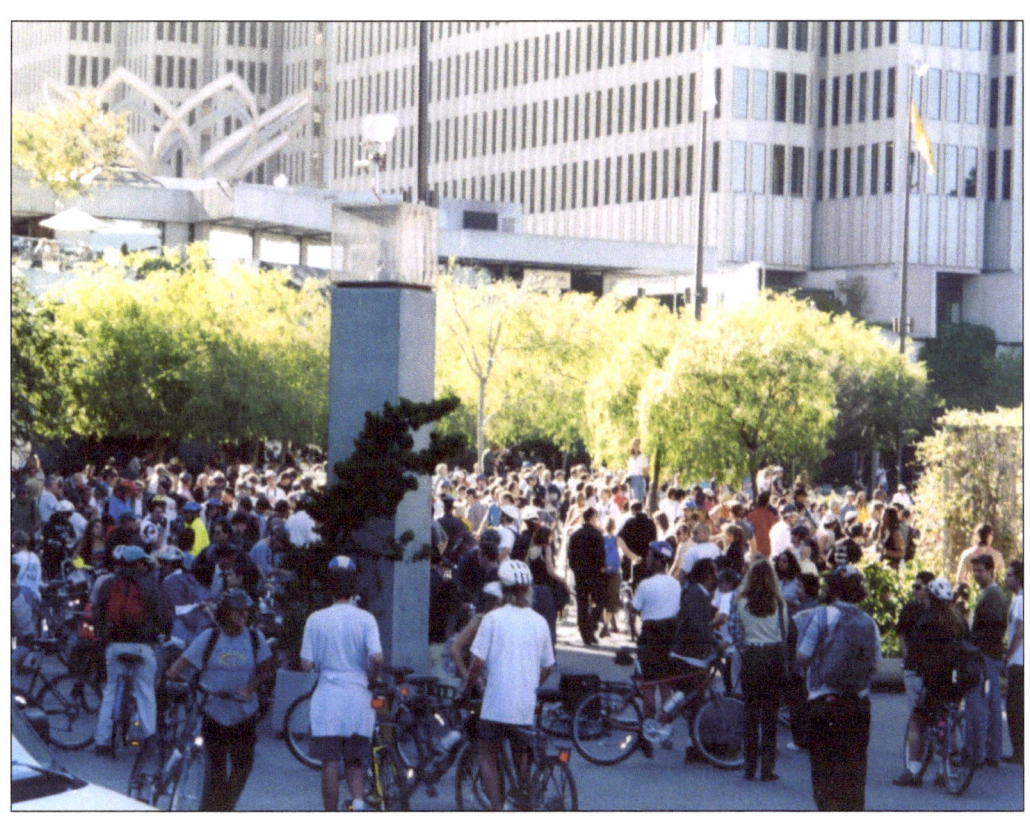

Critical Mass participants – Justin 'Pee Wee' Herman plaza, San Francisco

The original *Critical Mass* participants followed a San Francisco tradition of staging protests imbued with creativity and celebration. During the 1960s, the terms 'be-in' and 'happening' were coined here to describe this festival like feel to a gathering. *Critical Mass* began in the same manner. It grew to nearly 200 riders within six months and by its second anniversary ride in 1994, had nearly a thousand enthusiastic participants.[17]

In the early days, around 5 pm on the last Friday of the month, riders would begin congregating in Justin Herman plaza at the foot of Market Street, west of the San Francisco Ferry Building. A broad, flat, red brick area with several low concrete steps on its perimeter, the younger BMX[18] crowd soon became the opening entertainment as they spun around on the smooth bricks and launched impressive jumps from the steps.

---

17. In February 1993 a public art installation created by author and artist Chris Carlsson – depicting a human figure catapulting from a bike that has crashed into an open car door – was bolted to the ground at the foot of Market Street. The piece, entitled *"The Door Is Always Open,"* was removed by City authorities, but the story and message had already gone far and wide. See also cc@chriscarlsson.com
18. Bicycle motocross

By the time I arrived between 5 and 6 pm, there were usually several hundred cyclists milling around the plaza. Beautiful bikes and bike riding people in all directions! Many bikes were fantastic customized art pieces. Others were elaborately decorated and their riders likewise festooned in colorful custom made clothing. It was a whimsical looking scene with no shortage of clever and provocative messages scrawled on signs affixed to riders and bicycles. Riders rolled slowly through the group, making acquaintances, admiring the costumed wheels and wheel people. Many handed out information about bicycling related issues and events.

Just before 6 pm, the noise echoing off the adjacent Hyatt Regency hotel walls became a cacophony of loud voices and ringing bicycle bells. Catchy beats of musical favorites spanning decades were added by a contingent of bikers towing 'boom box' music players. People began fidgeting with helmets and gear. At 6 pm. the Ferry Building clock chimes rang out across the plaza and the chatter became a huge spontaneous cheer as bicyclists slowly began to roll up Market Street or along the Embarcadero.

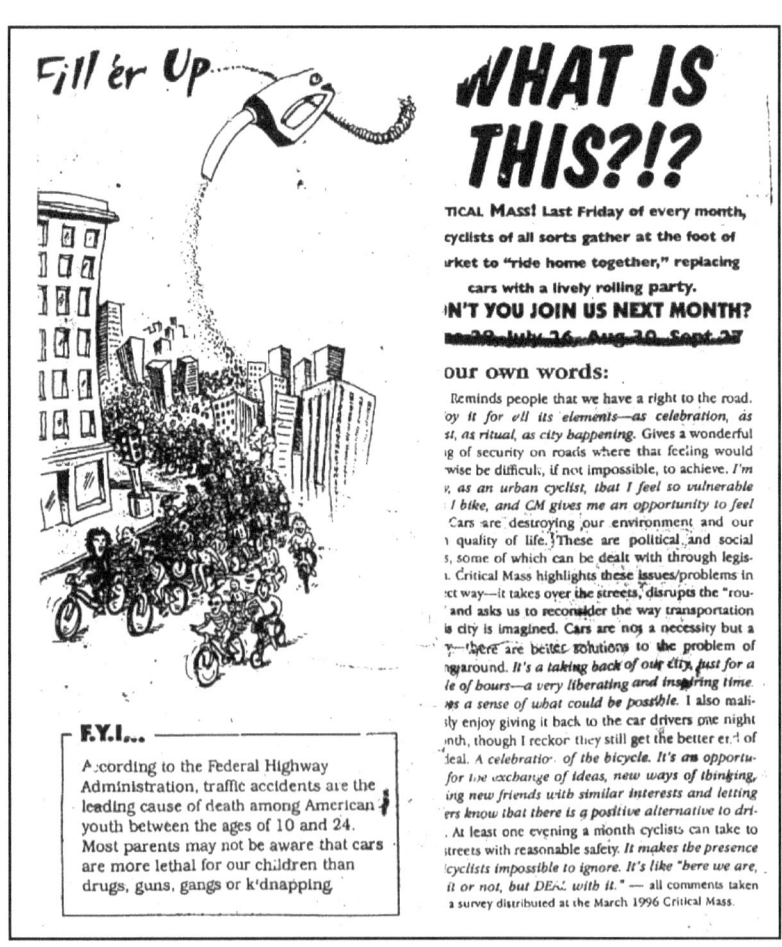

Early 1990s Critical Mass Flyer

In this early period, there were no actual ride leaders or police motorcycle escort. No one really knew where they were going and there was no predetermined destination. It didn't seem to matter much – different people took turns riding in the lead and eventually, the group would arrive somewhere familiar, like Dolores Park, the Palace of Fine Arts, Fort Point, eventually Ocean Beach and the Polo Fields cycle track in Golden Gate Park. Once a year, the group would trek across the Golden Gate Bridge to Sausalito. After reaching the destination, a gathering of the 'usuals' would ensue while the rest headed off into the night.

———————

Once the number of *Critical Mass* riders grew into the *thousands* a bigger picture became clear. Month after month I could see that some organizers and participants were focused on the opportunity for activism while others focused on the experience. It was impossible to ignore rides of this size which created a venue for a myriad of agendas. Since the free form structure allowed it, alternate 'leaders' were common, and different ride options were 'voted on' by shouts of support. Confusion among the participants was unavoidable and some who were 'just along for the ride' could realize that they weren't where they thought they would be. Nor was it all smiling pedestrians and curious motorists waving to the oddly dressed, noisy bicyclists rolling by. Some of those inconvenienced by the brief delays were truly *pissed off*. From time to time a driver or someone on foot would attempt to cross the stream of moving bicycles, only to have it take longer and be more dangerous than if they would have simply waited for the riders to pass. *Critical Mass* could be complicated!

Of course, the delays for pedestrians and drivers grew as the number of *Critical Mass* participants increased. Some months it was taking an impressive *ten* minutes or more for the group to pass through an intersection. It became apparent to many that something would emerge as a method of addressing the situation. City Hall and the SFPD were getting calls before, during and after the *Critical Mass* rides took place. As a group, cyclists were starting to feel noticed and listened to, but most City authorities and many others still viewed *Critical Mass* as a problem, not an opportunity.

For many of the riders, myself included, there was a desire to educate people – but we didn't want to cause fist fights! So, what evolved was the ingenious act of 'corking' an intersection, which can be defined as the act of temporarily blocking motor vehicle cross traffic in order to allow cyclists to pass and *remain in a group.* The 'corkers' were a group of cyclists who rode to the front of the group as they approached intersections and then stopped riding, remaining in a line in front of cars waiting to cross and allowing the larger group of cyclists to continue riding together. Some of the other riders would circulate among the blocked cars, handing drivers flyers explaining what *Critical Mass* was and listing the dates of future rides. If drivers began honking horns, corkers quickly displayed a sign reading *'Honk if you love bicycles!'* The corkers would then thread their way forward through the riders to the next intersection where the maneuver was needed. One might observe that the platoon of regular corkers were the backbone of the rides and kept things going as smoothly as they could. However, with a former Chief of Police, Frank Jordan, in the Mayor's office, it was inevitable that the Police Department would become involved.

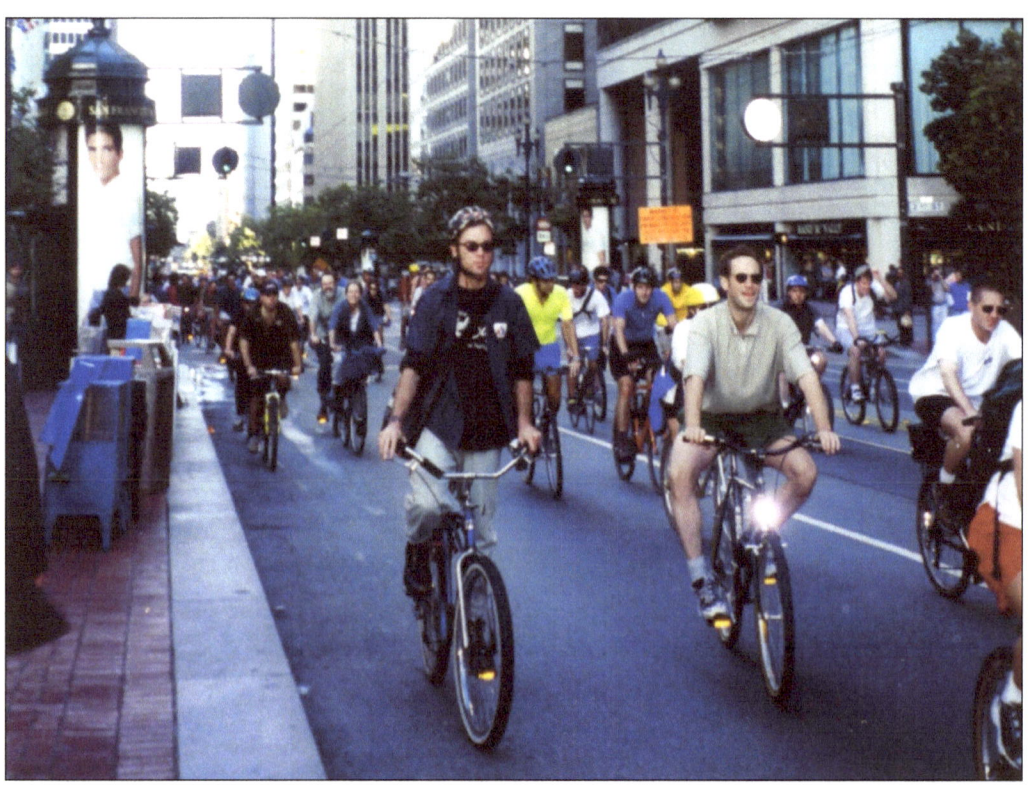

Critical Mass – Market Street, San Francisco

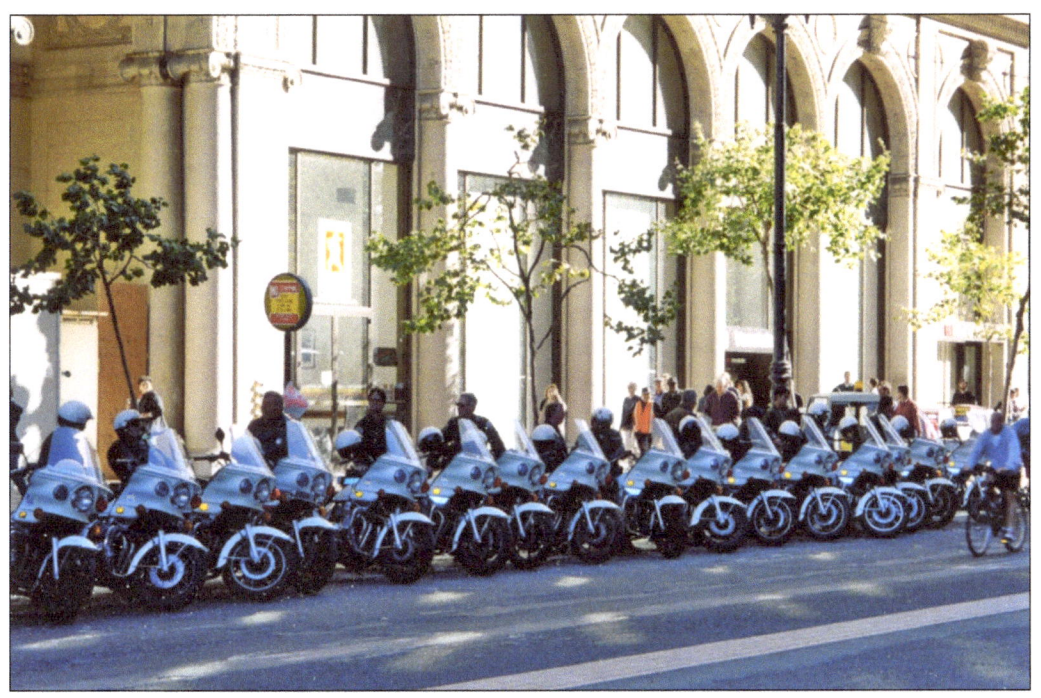

SFPD Motorcycle Unit waiting to escort Critical Mass – Market Street, San Francisco

Police officers directing Friday evening traffic on Market or Mission Streets downtown are a typical sight in San Francisco. Once a month when hundreds of cyclists approached the usual congested downtown intersections their task was simple. Traffic cops would stop car traffic and quickly wave the mass of cyclists through a few sequences of red lights. It was usually over in ten minutes or so. However, as *Critical Mass* grew, SFPD motorcycle officers were increasingly seen riding alongside the pack of cyclists. The months passed, the rides continued getting bigger, complaints increased and it became clear that City Hall was going to do something further. A dozen or more SFPD motorcycles began arriving at Justin Herman Plaza for *Critical Mass* before the ride got going at 6 pm.

There are varying opinions about the ultimate effect of the motorcycle police presence but the fact remains that initially they remained uninvolved observers. Throughout the months and years of my regular participation in *Critical Mass*, with the exception of July 25th, 1997, I never saw any confrontations – *ZERO!* 'Even the cops grooved with us' was a song lyric back in the 1960s and for *Critical Mass*, it still seemed true through the mid 1990s. When the clock chimed 6 pm, motorcycle cops donned their helmets, fired up their Harleys and quickly merged with the leading bicyclists. They constantly radioed to their fellow officers and relayed information about the rides' location, route and destination. A separate group of motorcycles often followed behind the main group of bike riders.

It continued to work systematically like this into the mid 1990s. The officers did the main amount of 'corking' wherever it was needed. It was an opportunity for them to conduct "rolling stop" maneuvers and minimize the slowing of motor vehicle traffic. *Critical Mass* was getting a police escort, not as a result of support for the ideas behind it, but because the Mayor and other authorities accepted that the ride had become a recurring event, reflecting a growing movement among cyclists of all stripes. City Hall had figured out that while they began to consider the numerous cycling-related issues that led to *Critical Mass*, they could also semi-manage the ongoing monthly ride events, which could go smoothly or create large scale *avoidable* problems, depending on how the details were addressed.

———

Willie Brown was elected Mayor in 1996 and the situation changed immediately. Unfortunately, he got directly involved and by the summer of 1997 *Critical Mass* riders witnessed things deteriorate dramatically. The Mayor ordered the motorcycle escorts to cease and as a result, the 'corkers' once again bore the burden of blocking pedestrians and cars while cyclists pedaled by. Only now, it could be as many as *a few thousand* cyclists, skaters and runners! The numbers of confrontations with those delayed grew. In June of 1997, during the annual *Critical Mass* ride to Sausalito, the Mayor himself was delayed in the resulting traffic congestion on the Golden Gate Bridge and *'went ballistic.'*

In his typical style, Brown attempted to commandeer the event in July, appearing at the foot of Market Street to announce the 'approved' route for *Critical Mass*. Most of the several thousand cyclists there could not hear him even if they were trying. The attempt to force agreement on the route was a publicity stunt failure! Wearing his Fedora and fur collared overcoat, the Mayor took the microphone to address the riders but was immediately and resoundingly shouted down and mocked by the crowd. He was silent and seething as his people escorted him away.

The antagonistic energy had escalated and made the situation worse. Riders began pedaling away in multiple directions, many simply falling in behind others, not realizing where they were going. The Mayor ordered the police into action and an entire block of downtown Montgomery Street was encircled by the police, trapping hundreds of cyclists. It was no surprise when tensions flared and cameras all around captured images of riders beaten and arrested in the effort to disperse the larger group. It was a Critical Mess! Perhaps like many riders who saw what happened but avoided arrest that evening, I left downtown feeling stunned, wondering what the hell had just happened and *why?*

All of the misdemeanor charges against the 110 cyclists arrested during this fiasco were dropped, and the City eventually paid damages and legal fees in at least one settlement with an injured cyclist. Cyclists and non cyclists all over the world were outraged at the heavy handed tactics. Over a thousand riders from all over the San Francisco Bay Area showed up for the August ride. 'We're not blocking traffic, we *ARE* traffic!' Hundreds more kept showing up in the following months. The message was loud and clear and had now been forged with completely avoidable violence. Mayor Brown attempted to blame the cyclists but could do nothing to engineer a shutdown of *Critical Mass*.

Joel Pomerantz, a cofounder, had called *Critical Mass* San Francisco's "defiant celebration" but in five years it had become much more. It had accomplished something and the events resonated everywhere. Mass bike ride events began happening all over the world! Despite Willie Brown, the rides in San Francisco continued and remained well attended. For many, they became obligatory. Most importantly, the City finally began developing a citywide comprehensive Bicycle Plan and the cycling community was given a 'place at the table.'

The following summer was designated as "Bike Summer 1998" in San Francisco and mainstream groups participating in the more structured events credited *Critical Mass* for "spotlighting" the important issues. However, *Critical Mass* offshoots and other events also began taking place in the late 1990s. Many cycling groups and individuals contributed to giving a stronger voice to the bicycling community as the City prepared its Bicycle Plan.

Predictably, Mayor Brown's successor, Gavin Newsom, changed policy soon after his election in 2004. The tenor of the City's dialogue with the cycling community shifted. San Francisco's Bicycle Plan was approved by the Board of Supervisors the following year and outlined 60 projects. The City approved a revised plan in 2009 and began adding 34 miles of bike lanes to the 45 miles that existed in 2010.

The City's Municipal Transportation Agency also began to make other badly needed changes out on the streets, adding signage, bike racks and parking, access to transit, trail access, 'speed bumps,' raised medians and physical separations from autos. In some places motor vehicle traffic lanes have even been eliminated in favor of accommodating bicycles. As of 2022, the amount of 'high quality'[19] bike routes in San Francisco stands at 121miles, within a bicycle network totaling nearly 450 miles.[20]

Riding together among hundreds of cyclists is a spectacular opportunity to keep the activism going while celebrating the joy of bicycling. The tradition has stayed strong here and world wide. *Critical Mass* had its *32nd* anniversary ride in San Francisco on September 27, 2024 and now takes place regularly in over 300 cities around the planet! In the United States, dozens of cities from coast to coast have their own ongoing *Critical Mass* and bicycling advocacy events. 'Free – Together!', 'We *ARE* traffic!' and 'Honk if you love bicycles!' remain universal slogans here but *Critical Mass* regulars in Kathmandu, Nepal wax poetic. Their motto since beginning monthly rides in 2013 is 'Quake or shake, sunny or rainy, we have to flow with time for the next smile.'

---

19. The City defines this category as "bike paths, protected bikeways, neighborways and buffered bike lanes."
20. The San Francisco Municipal Transit Agency (SFMTA.com) and the SF Bike Coalition (SFBike.org) are important resources for information regarding route maps and bicycling in San Francisco.

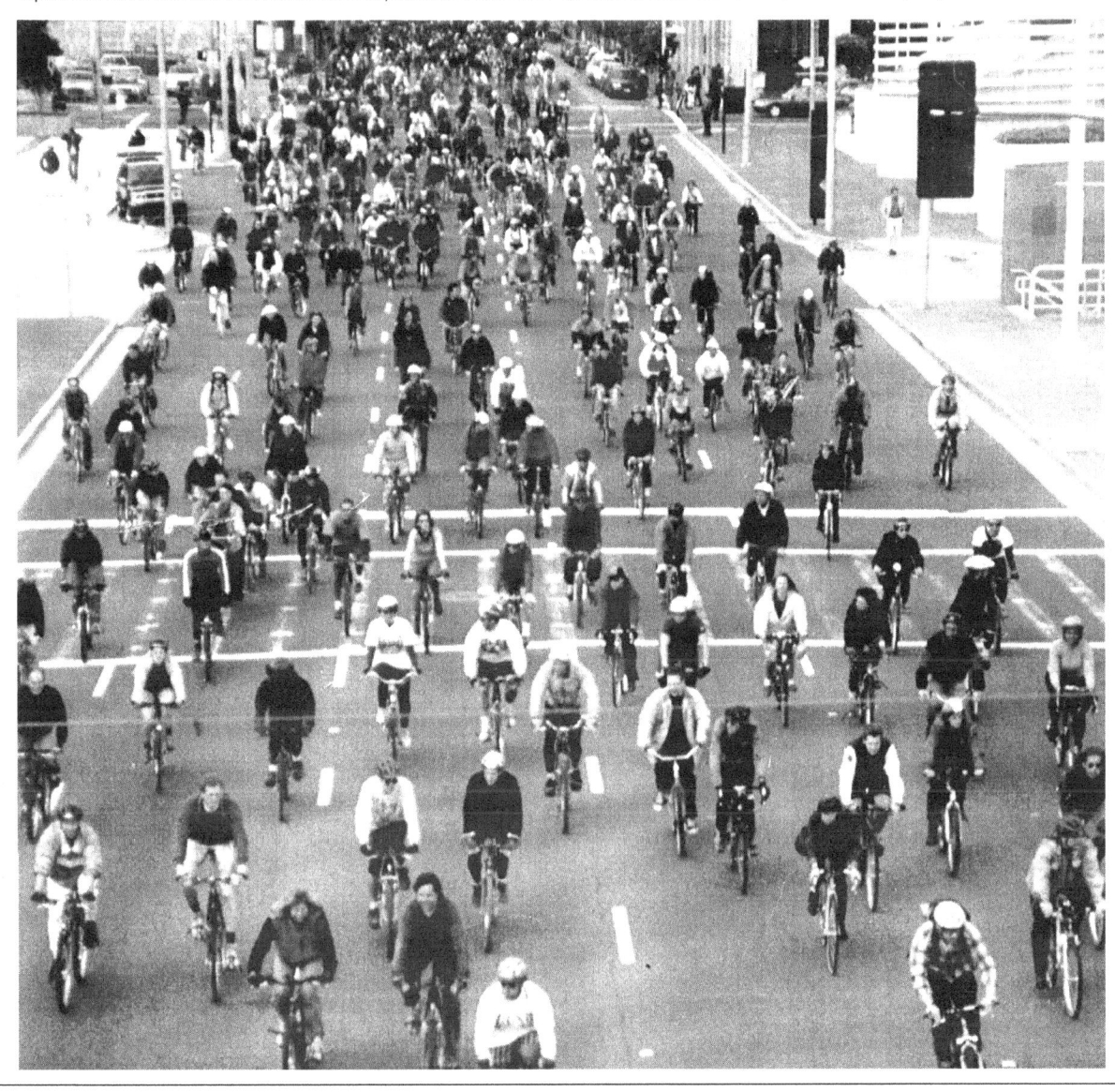

Critical Mass 3rd Anniversary Poster

*You boys ain't dressed for the weather...
Good Luck!*

– Gnarly-looking old 'roadie'
 Seen along Paradise Valley Road in Mount Rainier National Park

RAMROD - The Ride Around Mount Rainier in One Day (1993)

The 1990s continued a trend of exceptional years for cycling in the United States. The wave of popularity and public awareness that had surged in the 1980s showed no signs of reaching a crest anytime soon. Large scale 'benefit' rides and events such as *Critical Mass* became numerous. USA professionals were winning races in Europe and regional race events in the USA were exciting – attracting top international teams and well heeled sponsors. Bicycle sales were up. Cycling club membership was growing and recreational group rides were attracting hundreds, in some cases thousands, of participants. Weekly rides filled the calendars of cycling magazines and newsletters.

Of course, I was enjoying this modern heyday of cycling. I was feeling fit, having recovered significantly from my 1985 crash and hip fracture at The *World's Toughest Triathlon* eight years prior. I had two road bikes, a tandem, a track bike and a pre-WWII *Schwinn* – my 'balloon tire' cruiser. I rode them all – *regularly*. The hardware in my leg had been removed in 1989 and I'd bounced back quickly, getting on a bike just three weeks later.

By mid July of 1990, my form was such that I rode in that year's *Markleeville Death Ride* with my friend, Frank Varvaro. This 142 mile romp with 15,000 feet of climbing, later dubbed the *Tour of the California Alps*, has always been considered a pinnacle of alpine endurance cycling. Despite extremely harsh weather that day, Frank rode all *five* of the ride's tough Sierra passes in celebration of his 45th birthday. I managed *three* and we had a great time, overall. It was easy to build a tradition of riding in these tough, challenging cycling events together.

Living near Seattle, Washington, Frank became familiar with other premier endurance rides in the Pacific Northwest. The 156 mile *Ride Around Mount Rainier in One Day (RAMROD)* was one of them. Held annually in July, we 'set our sights' on riding the 10th annual *RAMROD* together in the summer of 1993. With 10,000 feet of climbing, it would be another feat of strength and endurance, a test of training and a *cyclist's resolve* – the ability to persevere and overcome obstacles. Little did I know how *much* of a test!

As its name suggests, the *RAMROD* course circumscribes the 14,411 foot high Mount Rainier. Sponsored by the Redmond Cycling Club, it was first staged as a 156 mile timed event in 1984 with a Start/Finish in Enumclaw – 62 miles northwest of Mount Rainier National Park's Nisqually entrance. That year, 45 of 52 riders finished. In 1993, our route proceeded from Enumclaw in a counterclockwise direction over the southern flank of the mountain, reaching an elevation of 5,400 feet at Paradise and climbing over the 4,700-foot Cayuse Pass before a final fifty mile descent back to Enumclaw.

Looking at the course profile, the 1993 *RAMROD* seemed pretty straight forward as endurance rides go. Basically, it consisted of one mountain – two passes with a 'bump' in between. The first climb, from the National Park entrance at Nisqually to Inspiration Pt. and Paradise, included some 3,400 feet of elevation gain over 18 miles, with 600 of those feet gained in the last two miles. The second big climb, over the 4,700 foot high Cayuse Pass, gained 2,500 feet of elevation in nine miles. The much shorter 'bump' in between was the three mile long 400 foot climb over Backbone Ridge.

The popularity of the ride had grown steadily in the late 1980s and by 1993 there were over 600 participants. In 1991, great weather and a shortened 152 mile route contributed to the first and only sub-seven hour finish time. By 1999, the National Park Service had requested that the timing of riders be discontinued and in 2001 there were 750 riders. A lottery system now caps the number of riders at 800 and the four mile loop to the Paradise Inn is no longer included. Regardless, tickets for the *RAMROD* remain immensely popular and are routinely resold at well above face value. Even Greg LeMond, the USA's first and *three* time *Tour de France* winner, made an appearance in 2004.

Once Frank and I decided to do the 1993 ride we proceeded to convince two other riding buddies to make it a group of four. Over the years, I had logged many miles with another longtime friend Shawn Ridley and the same was true for Frank and his Redmond

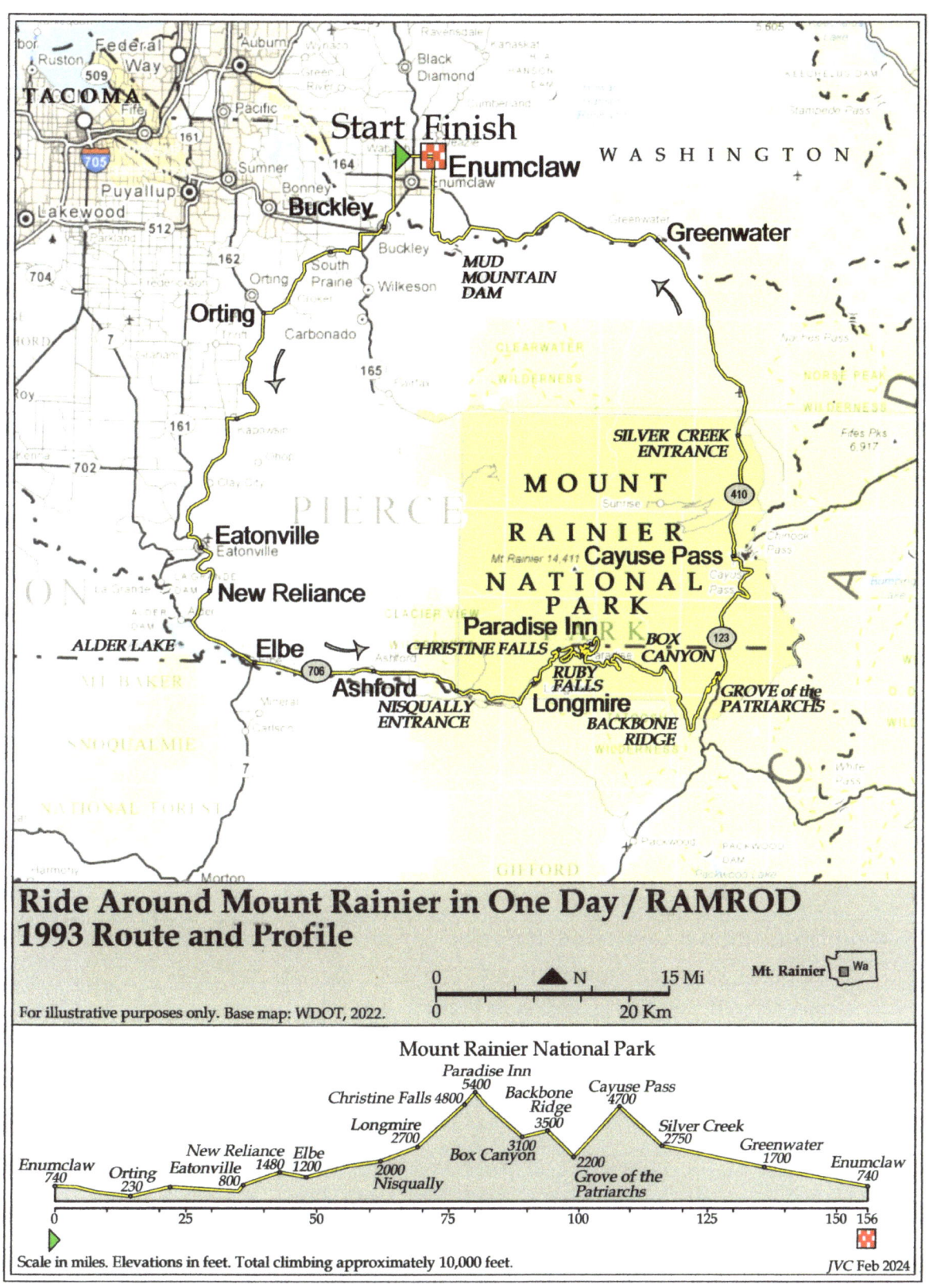

riding partner, Mike Roark. Both were game for the challenge and we all prepared ourselves during the first half of the year. I bought that year's *third* set of new tires in early July and Frank reminded us to bring decent raingear. Though the weather had been good during the previous editions, it would be no surprise if summer storms blew up over the mountain. I imagined a short, afternoon thundershower and would soon learn a hard lesson... Instead of actual raingear, I opted for aerosol waterproofing.

Mid July arrived and Shawn, his wife Sydney and I made the trek from California to Frank's place in Redmond, Washington over two days – stopping for the night in far northern California near Castle Crags and riding our bikes to the timberline of the majestic 14,162 foot high Mt. Shasta early the following morning. The 14 mile long Everitt Memorial Highway meanders its way up the flank of Mt. Rainier's southern Cascadian cousin, climbing about 4,500 feet from Mt. Shasta City to the old Ski Bowl trailhead where the road terminates at an elevation of 8,000 feet.

Rough pavement and the average six percent grade made it a steady, tough grind but the clear morning air and expansive high elevation views to the southwest were stunning. The temperature was perfect for a fast descent but the payback for all that climbing was not 'in the cards' for us. Numerous cattle crossings and wide separations in the asphalt pavement made it impossible to gain any real momentum on our return ride downhill to Mt. Shasta City.

We arrived at Frank's place in Redmond Thursday evening. The following day Shawn and I checked our bikes and organized our riding gear. I sprayed all of my outer cycling clothes with the waterproofing, which smelled like solvent. I had doubts about whether this malodorous stuff would work as I hung my 'raingear' outside Frank's garage to dry. Later that afternoon, we met Mike Roark and after one of Frank's pasta dinners, headed to the Marymoor velodrome to watch the Friday night events. The combination of higher latitude, summer season and daylight savings time made it a perfect night for racing – the action at the outdoor track continued until late in the evening.

On Saturday morning we were up early to load the four bikes and gear before starting the drive to Enumclaw, about 45 miles to the south. As we drove the light of dawn revealed a panoramic view of the imposing and magnificent, grey-shrouded Mt. Rainier directly ahead. Through the windshield of Frank's Bronco the mountain was dark and dominated the landscape almost the entire way to our start point. The weather was cool, humid and unsettled. I was glad I'd worn several layers and 'waterproofed' my jacket and tights.

We arrived in Enumclaw High School and rolled out around 7:30 am. After crossing the bridge over the White River to Buckley, we began a gradual descent to South Prairie and then continued downhill to the lowest point of the ride near Orting, at an elevation of 230 feet. It was forty minutes or so of fast, fun and flat 'valley riding,' complete with a cool, misty morning fog hovering over the ponds and low lying fields.

The second hour felt similar as we now rode gradually uphill along the Puyallup River to Electron and past Lake Kapowsin to our first stop in Eatonville. From there we headed into the forest towards Alder Lake, east to Elbe and along the Nisqually River, gradually uphill past Ashford to the National Park entrance at Nisqually. We had reached the 62 mile mark and an elevation of 2,000 feet in just over three hours.

Before we began the steady eighteen mile grind up to Paradise at 5,400 feet, it was time for a short rest and repair stop. The first 62 miles had been great – we all felt good and kept our pace high – but somewhere along the line I had broken a spoke and needed to take care of it there at Nisqually. Fortunately, it was on the *non*-freewheel side of the rear wheel. Mike and I flipped the bike upside down, removed the spoke and retrued the wheel while Frank and Shawn ate snacks and jokingly attempted to supervise.

The gradual, steady uphill along Paradise Valley Rd. to Longmire was next. There, we started the long steeper climb to Paradise and got the first inkling of the cold, wet weather ahead. The clouds were darkening quickly. Eventually, we caught up to a gnarly looking old 'roadie,' sporting shoe covers and a hooded, yellow rain slicker, tooling up the road in an easy low gear. I could smell hot coffee. His custom touring bike had front and rear panniers and I could see that his metal thermos was open and within easy reach. We greeted him like a respected elder and I wondered how much weight he was pulling as we rode slowly passed. He raised his coffee cup as if to toast us and nodded, uttering words that I remember as well as his Eddy Merckx-era Molteni cycling cap, *"You boys ain't dressed for the weather... Good Luck!"*

We chuckled but his observation was spot-on. As we gained elevation and worked harder, the temperature dropped steadily and the sky overhead turned black. I started thinking about that yellow rain slicker and wondering about my waterproofing. We passed Christine Falls Bridge and finally reached Ruby Falls at Mile 78. A cold rain, wind gusts and snow flurries commenced as we climbed two more steep miles to the Paradise Inn, arriving around noon. Our clothes were damp and it was freezing out but we had reached the highest elevation of the ride – covering eighty miles in roughly four and a half hours.

Outside the Inn the parking lot was a sea of bicycles. Inside, droves of cyclists crowded the dining room's gigantic stone fireplace, where a roaring blaze burned. We did our best to warm up a bit but it was too noisy to do much more than drink hot coffee and get going.

The weather had become severe and the rapid descent back towards Inspiration Pt. was not only steep but miserably cold. The snow flurries turned to steady rain as we made the six mile descent along Stevens Canyon Rd. Sections of cracked pavement and iron grated drains across the road didn't help matters. Moisture hung in the air and any possible views were obscured by the heavy, dark clouds. We passed Reflection Lakes, Louise Lake, and Bench Lake and rolled downhill along steep, vertically sided roads, cut directly into bare rock. The heavy braking through tunnels and steep switchback turns stiffened my hands. At Box Canyon we began the nearly five mile climb over Backbone Ridge and finally arrived at Mile 99, the Grove of the Patriarchs. The old roadie had been right… we were stone cold and our kits were soaked. My spray-on 'waterproofing' was a complete fail!

The next hour or so was spent enduring a brutal nine mile long, 2,500 foot climb over Cayuse Pass – as the weather worsened even further! The old roadie was affirmed yet again. A heavy downpour began falling as we made it over the pass and began a nightmarish, gusty, slick and sweeping descent along the Mather Memorial Highway. It was the kind of rain that hurts when it hits you, pelting rain that forces you to turn your face away and ride with your hands on the brake levers. At Silver Creek, the road flattened out but we were given another twenty mile long drenching as we rolled along the White River on the descent to Greenwater.

There, saturated, after enduring nearly two hours and 30 miles of what is still described as the *RAMROD's* "worst weather ever experienced," we bailed to the 'sag wagon.'

We missed out on the Mud Mountain Dam Rd. descent and the last 20 miles or so to the event finish but it turned out we weren't the only ones. The intense rain continued all the way to Enumclaw that afternoon and many others took advantage of the 'sag wagon' vans steadily shuttling riders and their bikes back to the Start/Finish in Enumclaw. Only 508 riders were able to complete the 1993 ride. Regardless, riding 136 miles in less than eight hours – with that much climbing and under those conditions – was a huge accomplishment for each one in our group. It was, without a doubt, one of the toughest rides that I'd ever done.

I was still pouring water out of my shoes or too exhausted to notice that Frank managed to get each of us *RAMROD* finisher's pins. He gave them to us later. We had come up twenty miles short but it didn't matter, we accomplished the *RAMROD* in a way that we didn't expect – by enduring the extreme weather. As I cleaned up our bikes the next morning I thought about what we had done and the old roadie whose observation about our clothing turned out to be such an understatement. His entire approach to the ride illustrated the lesson: *Situations can be deceiving and reality, much different than what it seems to be. Conditions can change in a flash. Be ready, since things often don't go exactly as planned and remember – Aerosol waterproofing is useless in a steady downpour!*

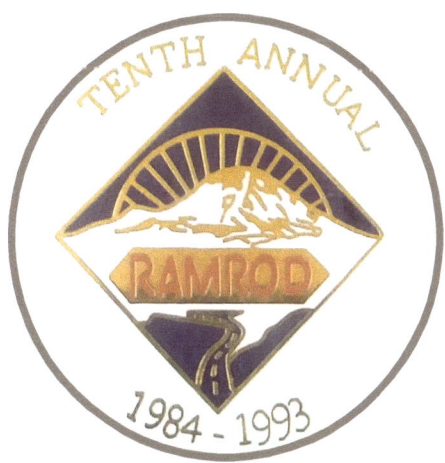

RAMROD 10th Anniversary finisher's pin

Wow! 200 Miles is a long ways to ride in a day

– 'Celtic huntress'
Seen along Westside Highway outside of Vader, WA

STP - Seattle to Portland (1994)

The 206 mile ride from *Seattle to Portland (STP)* in 1994 was a perfect contrast to my previous year's storm shortened attempt to complete the *Ride Around Mount Rainier in One Day (RAMROD)*. My friend Frank Varvaro lived near Seattle and had learned about *STP*, staged by the Cascade Bike Club each summer. Early in the year, he invited me to trek north from San Francisco for the 15th anniversary ride.

STP has been taking place since 1979. It was first staged as a time trial[21] and after being shortened in 1980 due to the eruption of Mount St. Helens, became a very popular and well supported long distance recreational ride. Each year several thousand cyclists spend an overnight somewhere near Centralia and complete the distance over two days. I was intrigued at the challenge but 200 miles seemed like a long distance to ride – with or without an overnight. I'd done multi day rides but never a 'double century.'[22]

Being a cyclist *and* a cartographer has its advantages, though. Soon I had studied the course and convinced myself that *STP* could be ridden in *one* day – on my tandem. The meandering route began at the University of Washington soccer stadium and continued south from Seattle, generally along Interstate Highway 5. A significant part of the ride was parallel to the railroad alignment. The terrain would range from urban and industrial to small town and rural. The topography appeared to be mostly flat, gentle and rolling, with a profile that included just 30 miles or so of 'uphill.' The biggest climb was near Puyallup, where 440 ft. of elevation is gained in about three miles. It would be a perfect opportunity to take my beloved *Santana Marathon* on its longest jaunt ever. I immediately talked to my longtime friend and fellow cyclist, Tom Mikkelsen, to gauge his interest in teaming up for the event.

My *Santana* tandem such a comfortable, fun bike to ride! A 1979 – with beautiful metallic, midnight blue paint, an extra strong *Tange* front fork, rear rack and disc brake. I set it up as a 'day tripper' with 28 mm tires on 40 spoke wheels, making

---

21. A time trial is an individual or team race against the clock.
22. A double century is a 200 mile or 200 kilometer ride.

it lighter and theoretically quicker than most touring tandems. The previous owner had installed an expensive, *Campagnolo Record* crankset, custom drilled to accept a third chainring. I coupled its 36, 46 and 54 tooth chainrings with 13 to 30 tooth freewheel gears on the rear hub and away I went... The shorter, 170 mm crank arms made it easy to accelerate quickly.

The *Santana's* wide gearing provided for comfortable pedaling no matter who was in back. I loved riding this bike from the moment it was mine! By 1994, there had been many 'picnic' rides with girlfriends but Tom and I were superbly matched on the bike. Being about the same height, weight and strength allowed us to alternate riding in front without even needing to adjust the saddle positions. We had begun taking turns as 'captain' and 'stoker' while we breezed around the Bay Area on flat century rides in five hours. Not surprisingly, Tom agreed to my scheme of doing *STP* in one day on the *Santana*.

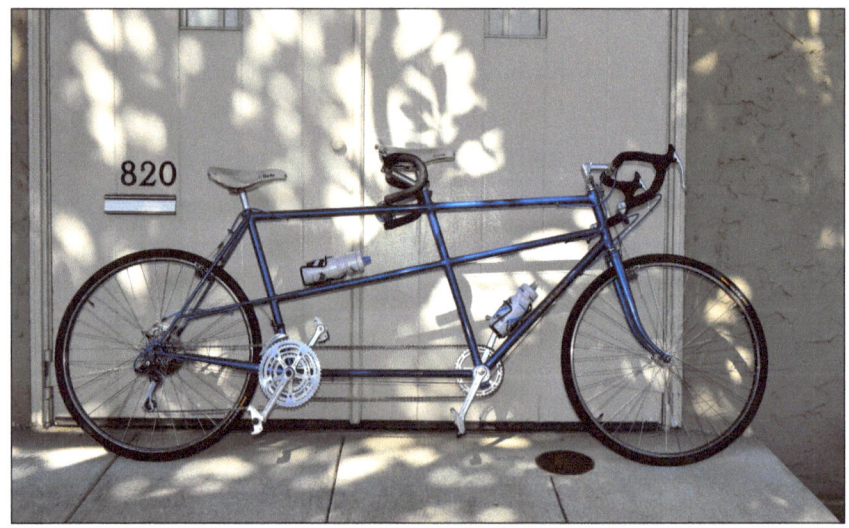

'Midnight' – aka my **1979 *Santana Marathon* tandem**

Long distance cycling events are not just about strength and endurance. They also require good bike handling skills and a measure of patience for riding in large groups. *STP* turns out to be one of the ten biggest rides in the United States – *year after* year. In 1989 there were 10,000 participants! In recent years, nearly 25 percent of the cyclists complete the ride in one day. Imagine riding through the middle of western Washington during the middle of a summer day with several thousand bicycle riders

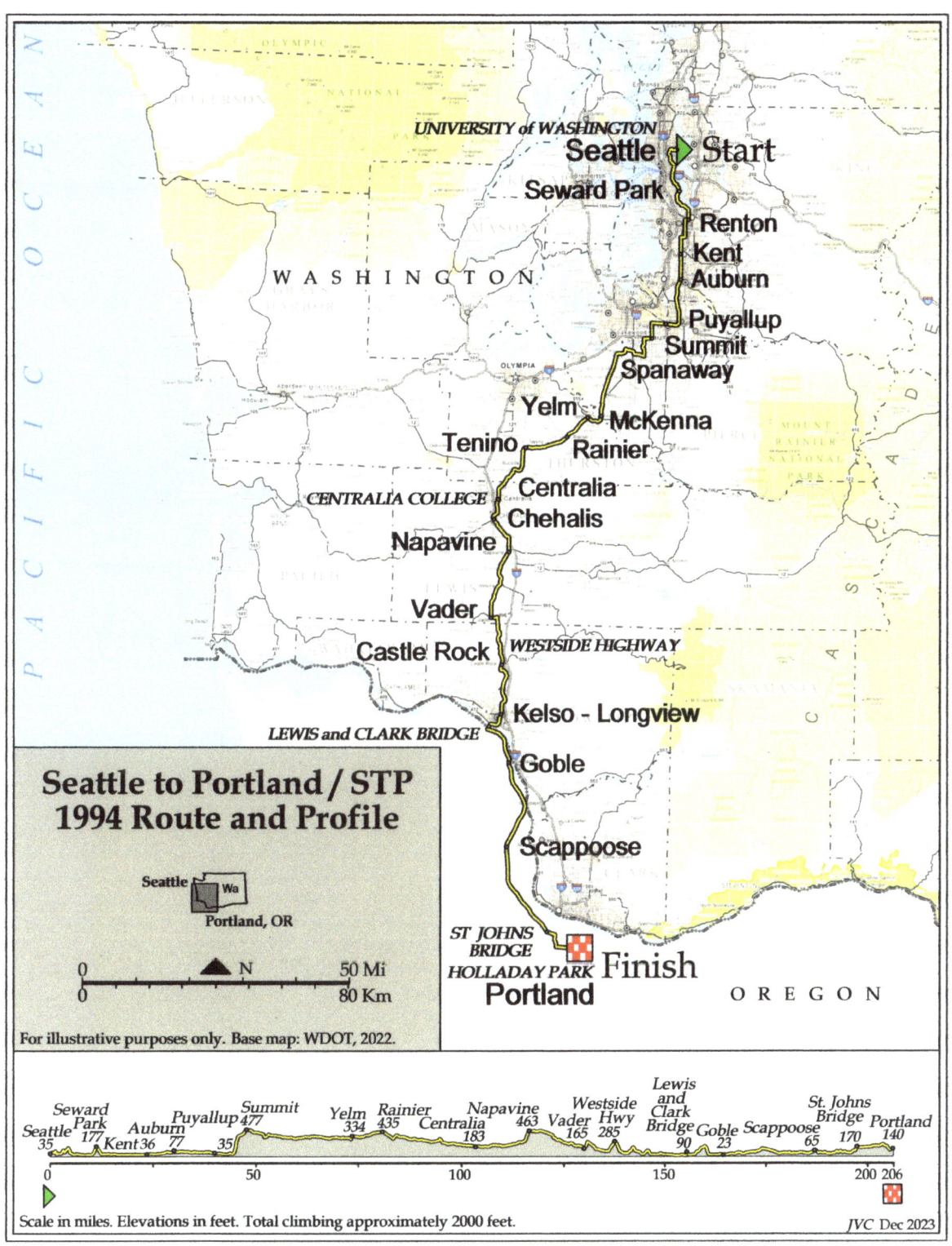

on the same roads, all heading to the same destination. As one might expect, many of the things that *can* happen to bicyclists are bound to happen... simply a function of the numbers.

It's both exhilarating and challenging to ride in a large group – or even stressful if you're not used to it. Riding the *Santana* in many of the Bay Area century rides, Tom and I had developed the sufficient skills and confidence needed to maneuver a weighty, long wheelbase tandem through waves of slow moving cyclists. The 1994 *STP* would be an *anniversary* ride with many first time participants – including us. It was a given that we would have plenty of opportunities to test both our patience and *our* bike handling skills.

Once I had registered for the event Tom and I got busy training. We fitted my bike rack onto his car and began staging longer training rides in California's Sierra Nevada foothills and San Joaquin Valley. Mid June rolled around and we made preparations for the trip to Redmond, Washington. Frank's buddy Mike would also be joining us, making it a quartet. A perfect plan for the big day emerged – Frank recruited his daughter Mary to drive his Bronco on a parallel route south and rendezvous with us at specific locations along the way, providing any extra support we might need and, of course, the vehicle for our return from Portland after a guaranteed 'long day in the saddle.'

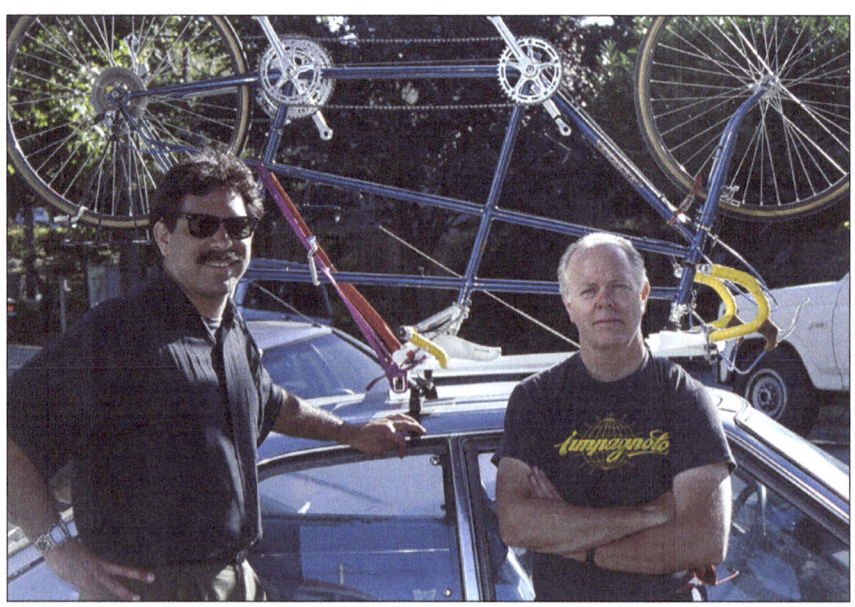

Heading to Seattle, June 1994 (with Tom Mikkelsen)

Tom and I left San Francisco the Thursday before *STP* and drove north on Interstate Highway 5, checking the bike at each gasoline stop to make sure it remained secure. My unconventional roof rack was designed to hold a bicycle positioned 'upside down,' attached mainly at the handlebars and front saddle. We had rigged additional tie downs for the longer, heavier tandem frame. It must have looked a bit odd... but it worked.

The years have rendered some details of the trip to Redmond a tad fuzzy. It was definitely Mexican food for dinner but was it an overnight in Yreka, California or Corvallis, Oregon? Wherever it was, the espresso stops the next day did the trick and we arrived at Frank's place early Friday afternoon. Later, after unloading and getting the Santana situated for Saturday's ride, we settled in to enjoy Frank's pasta dinner and French wine, followed by a viewing of Joël Santoni's classic 1974 film, *'La Course en Tête,'* about cycling's great Belgian star, Eddy Merckx. Tom had brought his personal copy of the video along just for the occasion. The cycling *repartee* was premium and though the combination of daylight savings time and high latitude summer delayed sunset until almost 10 pm, the anticipation of an early start meant calling it a night much sooner than we preferred.

The following morning we did our best to get going and arrived at the stadium parking lot close to 6 am. Day was dawning and, remarkably, well over a thousand riders were already out on the road ahead of us. A steady stream of blinking bicycle tail lights was moving through the campus towards Portage Bay and Lake Washington. Many *two* day participants were still arriving to register but luckily we breezed through the process. We were a bit 'behind schedule' and among the last of the *one* day riders to depart.

The sky was dark and grey as we rolled out, eventually clearing to reveal a beautiful blue sky punctuated with billowy cumulus clouds. The light breezes that developed later were mostly behind us and we couldn't have asked for better overall riding conditions. The weather would ultimately stand in stark contrast to that of the previous year's *RAMROD,* during which Frank and I endured hours of drenching in a pelting downpour under heavy, black clouds. *STP* felt different right away. It was going to be a pleasant day!

The first hour was a slow going, scenic cruise along the western shore of Lake Washington to Andrews Bay and Seward Park. If felt like a snail's pace though we were continually passing slower riders once we got started. Everybody loves a nice looking tandem, so it was also a fun, social part of the ride – albeit a little hectic – with riders two and three abreast cruising on two lane streets. Hour two was quite the opposite. I realized that we had caught and become imbedded in a continuous stream of groups ranging from twenty or so to several *hundred!* Somehow we managed to keep moving forward slowly along the flat, suburban and industrial thoroughfares. There were railroad crossings and long, straight arterials with 'cross traffic' and numerous traffic lights.[23]

The tedious riding continued past Renton, through Kent, Algona, and Pacific – all the way to Sumner. The industrial architecture was uninteresting and the scenery – repetitive of the commercial business corridors found in many US cities. From floor tiles, tires and Thai food to building materials, bulk pet supplies and housewares – you could get it *all* here. Finally, we emerged from the urban and industrial areas south of Seattle into the countryside. The terrain began to remind me of valleys and woodlands in the San Francisco Bay Area.

The groups of *STP* cyclists now casually formed three steady streams of riders – a slower line to the right, a middle line for most others and a third one to the left, for those wanting to pass or proceed at a faster pace. It all seemed pretty civilized but I was definitely using my bell more than usual. It was my 'dumb bell for the '*dumbbells'* and there seemed to be a lot of them that day. The railroad crossings created bottlenecks for everyone, each pair of tracks forced riders to slow down, cross and then speed up to regain their momentum.

During hour three we reached the so called 'big hill,' a three mile climb out of Puyallup. Here we were – two 80 kg men on a 20 kg bike – threading our way uphill about 440 feet, steadily spinning and steering through the short, steep inclines past our mostly slower moving compatriots. At the crest we continued along the flats to Spanaway, then south through Lewis-McChord joint military base over the rough roads to Roy and on to Yelm.

---

23. The full *STP* route includes over *35* railroad crossings.

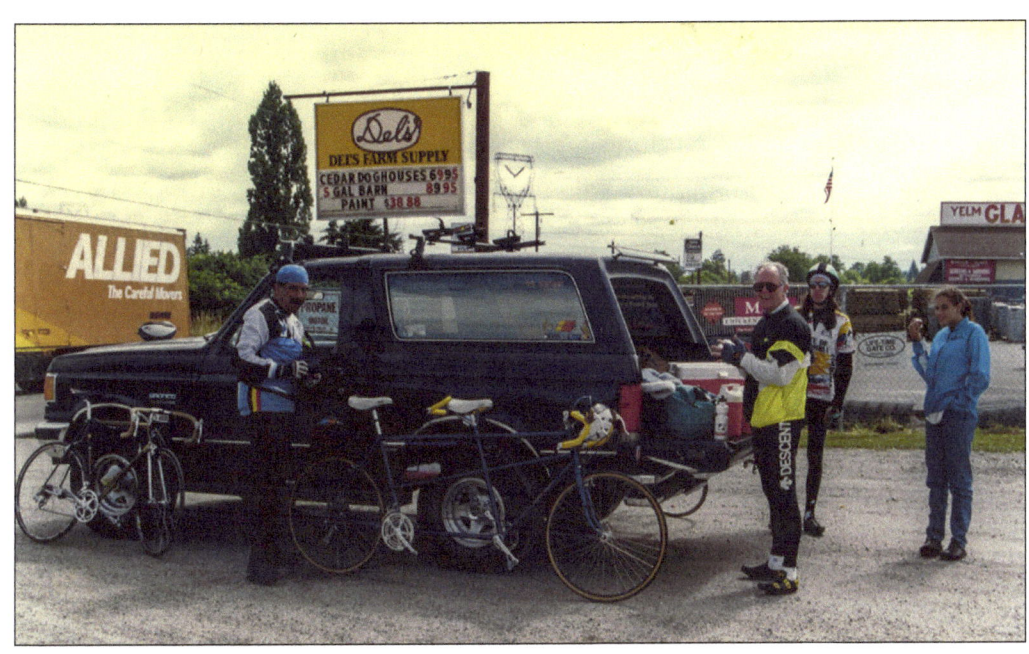

STP – Off the bike for a break at Yelm

The constant congestion continued... with an uptick in the number of 'knuckleheads' trying to speed through the group along the narrower segments. Others stopped suddenly for no apparent reason, or stood chatting in the roadway at water stops and intersections. An amazing number of riders made awkward maneuvers without paying attention! As we began hour four and entered the wooded bike trail at Yelm 'bicyclists behaving badly' suddenly met 'traffic furniture.' Four foot high heavy wooden posts were located mid path at street crossings. Fourteen miles later, we reached Tenino and continued on city streets to Mile 103 – *STP's* halfway point at Centralia College. It was 11:30 am.

Overall, the first half of the ride had been mostly flat and congested – a long and tedious group ride – nothing too strenuous. The pace felt sluggish though we'd been passing other riders for the entire five and a half hours. Nevertheless, we were mostly having great fun. There were no flat tires or mechanical problems. The weather had been grey to blue but pleasant and mild – the rural landscapes and pastoral scenery looked picturesque and stunning – like works of the 19th century French Barbizon School painters, Corot, Rousseau and others... only there were bicycles everywhere.

The skies turned bluer and the afternoon temperature became warmer but once we left Centralia the most noticeable change was a welcome *decrease* in the number of riders. The two day crowd was done for the day and the *one* day cyclists now shrank into manageable groups of tens or even a hundred, as opposed to the steady stream of riders we encountered all morning. It was much easier to navigate through the pack as we rode on to Chehalis, reached the second 'big hill' and gained about 200 feet of elevation in a short climb to Napavine, then continued through Winlock to Vader.

Perhaps there's one on *every* memorable ride! A lone cyclist – who appears at an unlikely moment, for no apparent reason – seemingly out of place or oddly equipped but nonetheless able to ride along with the group or sometimes easily past them. Just as we began the short uphill out of Vader, there she was – a young woman wearing a suede leather vest and green dress, her long curly red hair flying back as she made the turn from a side street and temporarily joined our bunch. Her front basket was full of cut flowers. Looking like a Celtic huntress, she stood on the pedals of her old three speed *English Racer* and cruised by the new bikes and *STP* riders sporting the latest cycling clothes and bike gear.

"Nice bike, Mister!" She said, as she rolled past, alongside Tom and me. I was still *thirty nine* but suddenly I felt *forty*...

"Thanks," I replied dryly, "You've got yourself a nice old *Raleigh* there, too."

"Used to be my dad's... Hey – where's everybody goin,' anyway?" She was steadily pulling away, up the gradual incline. I sensed that she was curious but didn't really care.

"Seattle to Portland... 200 miles," Tom called out to her.

"Wow! 200 miles is a long ways to ride in a day." Her voice trailed off in the distance, affirming in a moment what I'd been certain of since spring. Tom and I had trained up to 120 miles or so all year but nothing close to a full *200* miles. We still had quite a "long ways" to go. The 'Celtic huntress' danced away on the pedals like *Alberto Contador*[24] in sandals, disappearing up the road – never to be seen again.

---

24. Spaniard Alberto Contador is a multiple Grand Tour winner and Tour de France champion known for his dance-like style of climbing.

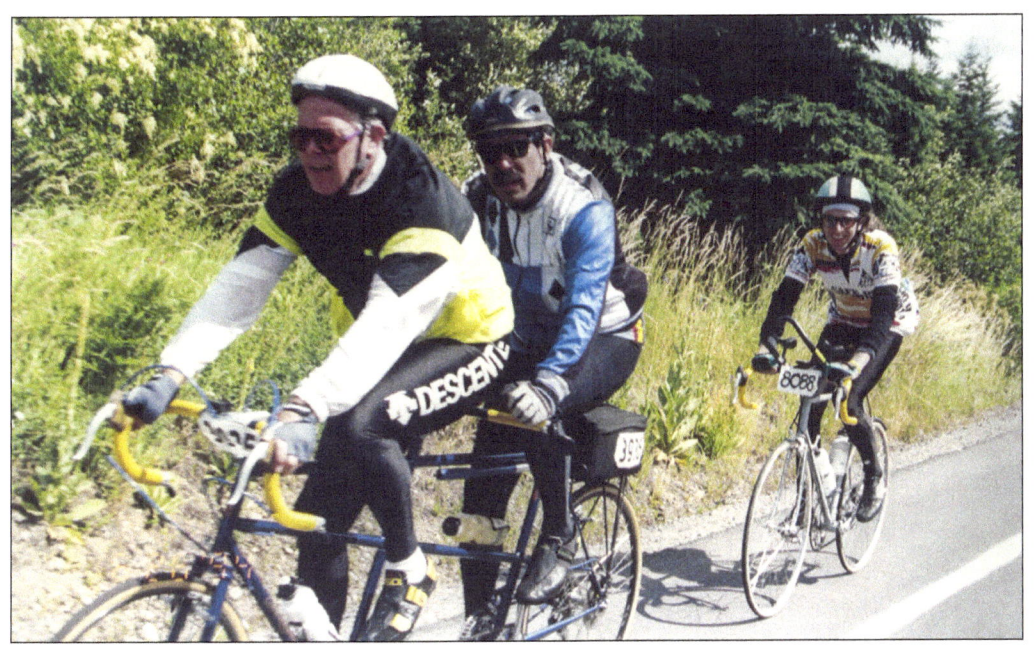

STP – Working our way through Washington

Yes, 200 miles is a long way to ride in one day but we were doing it – *sans incident*.[25] During hour seven, we had moved forward quickly through the smaller groups, continually passing other riders steadily along the flat bike path to Vader and Westside Highway to Castle Rock. It seemed that our 'late start' had put us in a perfect position now at 2 pm. With our faster pace and bigger gaps between cyclists along the flat country roads we made good time all the way to Kelso-Longview.

The *one* day *STP* ride is interesting in that, although technically a recreational event, some ride it as a personal time trial. A definite subset of the *one* day participants races against the clock attempting to finish in less than ten to twelve hours. This particular year, 1994, two young men on a fixed gear tandem completed the ride in amazingly fast time of 9.5 hours! However, being in the realm of fit, middle aged working men, Tom and I had 'set our sights' on 11 to 12 hours. We were doing a decent job making up for the slower first half of the ride, nevertheless, we were beginning hour *ten* and about to lose some time at Longview as we crossed the Lewis and Clark Bridge over the Columbia River into Oregon.

There was a transition to riding the highway 'shoulder' as we approached the causeway leading to the 1.5 mile long *two lane* cantilever bridge. Opened in 1930 and initially built as a private

---

25. Translated as *without incident.*

toll bridge, the structure was designed by Joseph Strauss, of Golden Gate Bridge fame, and entered in the National Register of Historic Places in 1982. However, despite its pedigree and status, and unlike its 'Golden' sibling to the south, this particular landmark was not designed to accommodate either pedestrians or cyclists!

Getting across this bridge was a tense, hair-raising affair. It was easily the most *un*enjoyable part of the ride. There we were after riding 150 miles, confronting a final, three quarter mile long, low gear uphill grind, gaining 90 feet of elevation before an equally steep descent – along what is essentially a narrow, two lane *freeway* over a major river! Cars and trucks of all sizes whizzed by us in both directions, at speeds well over 60 miles an hour.

All cyclists were forced to ride in the narrow 'lane' adjacent to the steel side plates of the bridge structure. Besides having to avoid other riders slowing down on the steep incline, there were now patches of road debris directly in our path and bridge expansion joints to contend with. Steel cover plates were damaged or missing. It was 'slow going' for every cyclist. The gusty crosswinds and large road obstacles made it impossible pick up any speed on the descent into Rainier, Oregon. There, we began the last fifty miles along the Columbia River to Portland. I felt lucky – we'd gotten to Oregon safely – and not even a flat!

After the mildly harrowing Lewis and Clark Bridge experience and a wooded climb to Lindbergh we took our last 'off the bike' break at Goble – sincerely grateful for Mary and Frank, who had provided the perfect support in between official stops – an ice chest full of fruits, other food, drinks, coffee and *dry clothes!* With Mike rolling alongside we now began our last push and continued on, catching many individual riders. By the time we reached the two lane highway at St. Helens we were beginning hour eleven.

Maybe it's the endorphins or the anticipation of being finished soon but after ten or eleven hours of riding you truly begin feeling a 'second wind.' Something kicks in, you keep motoring along – and that's what we did. Mike took his now typical turns on the front and we all rolled through Scappoose along the incline to the St. John's Bridge and on into Portland. At last, we crossed our final sets of railroad tracks and continued through town reaching Holladay Park around 5:45 pm. All three of us were still smiling.

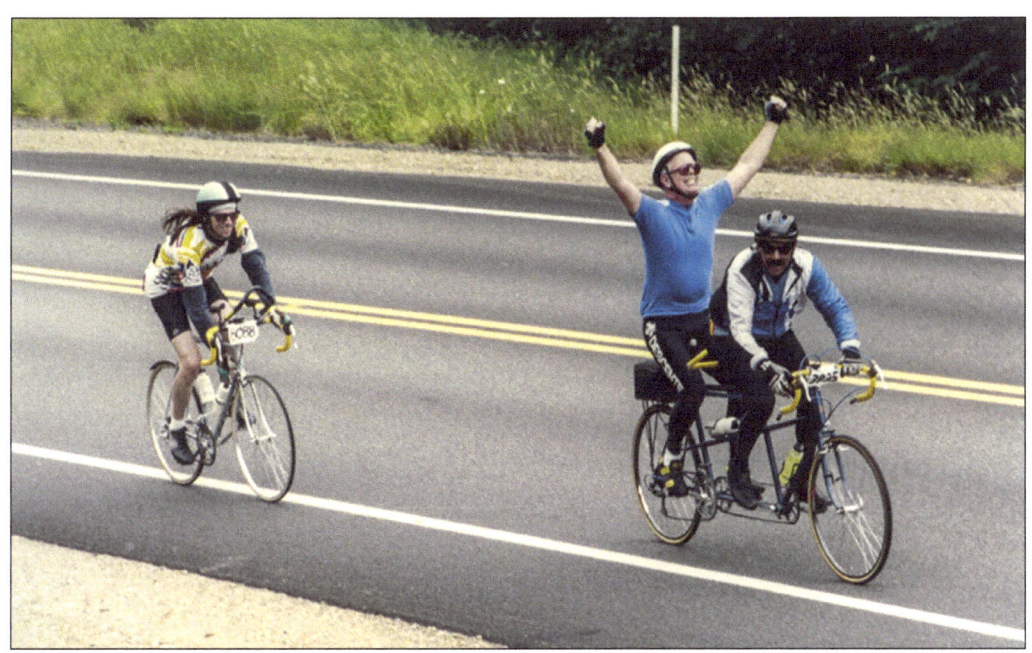

STP – Rolling into Portland

We unceremoniously loaded the bikes and gear into Frank's Bronco and headed for the *Riverplace Marina* and one of the riverfront Italian restaurants. All of us were predictably starving and a hearty, 'five star' dinner was enjoyed by all. Before long, we were elated, sated and feeling successful that we'd ridden 206 miles in 11 hours and 45 minutes.

After a round of espresso, we decided we'd better hit the road back to Seattle. Frank drove the first leg and before long we were back in Washington on Interstate 5 with Mary, Mike and Tom sound asleep in the back. Frank and I chatted about the long day's events. I was tired but not sleepy, or so I thought. About halfway back to Seattle I asked Frank if he wanted me to do some driving and he quickly agreed.

Soon I was speeding up the highway at 75 mph, the silent chauffeur to not three, but *four* sleeping cyclists. As I drove passed towns and cities we had been through over half a day earlier, I couldn't help but recall the young woman on the old *Raleigh* three speed. I could hear her voice in my mind, *"200 miles is a long ways to ride in a day."* Without a doubt she was right… it's a long way to d*rive* as well. It had taken *three* hours to get back to Seattle!

Our long day ended when we dropped Mike off and arrived back to Frank's house. After hot showers, a brandy 'nightcap' to salute our accomplishment was in order. We drank a toast to future cycling adventures and turned in for the night. Tom and I had to work on Monday and we were anticipating another marathon on the morrow – the 14 hour drive home.

Of course, Tom and I had lots of time to discuss *STP* and reflect on our experiences during the drive back to San Francisco. Now firmly based in reality, my perception of a riding a double century had completely changed. What I had thought would be simply a feat requiring strength and endurance was instead more a test of our patience and ability to immediately deal with the complete range of daylong interferences that we encountered.

It turned out that we were both plenty fit to ride a mostly flat 200 miles, and fully capable of navigating a tandem in a crowd but neither of us had anticipated the high volume of cycling 'knuckleheads,' route 'bottlenecks,' railroad tracks and road debris! A major part of the ride had required being alert and tense – ready for something unexpected. We had experienced zero bike problems – not even a flat tire – but it just wasn't a leisurely ride.

As I thought about it further it seemed that, once again, an epic bicycle ride had been something of a metaphor for life in general. *STP* held a lesson: though one's course might seem mostly level and easy in many ways – be prepared and ready – there can be plenty of moments when maneuvering among others might slow your progress – and moments when unavoidable obstacles appearing suddenly must be immediately overcome, by advancing over, under, around or through them. *STP* was a *life*-like journey.

_____

Completing the *STP* ride gave me something else. I'd fractured my hip pretty badly participating in the 1985 *World's Toughest Triathlon* almost nine years earlier and after enduring surgery and some complications in the aftermath, had returned to long distance cycling as one of my lifelong favorite outdoor activities. I had done many long rides since 1985 but *STP* symbolized a major turning point in my recovery. After 1994, whenever I found myself recounting the triathlon accident to others I began finishing my story with the words: "… but I never rode my bike *200* miles in one day until *after* I broke my hip."

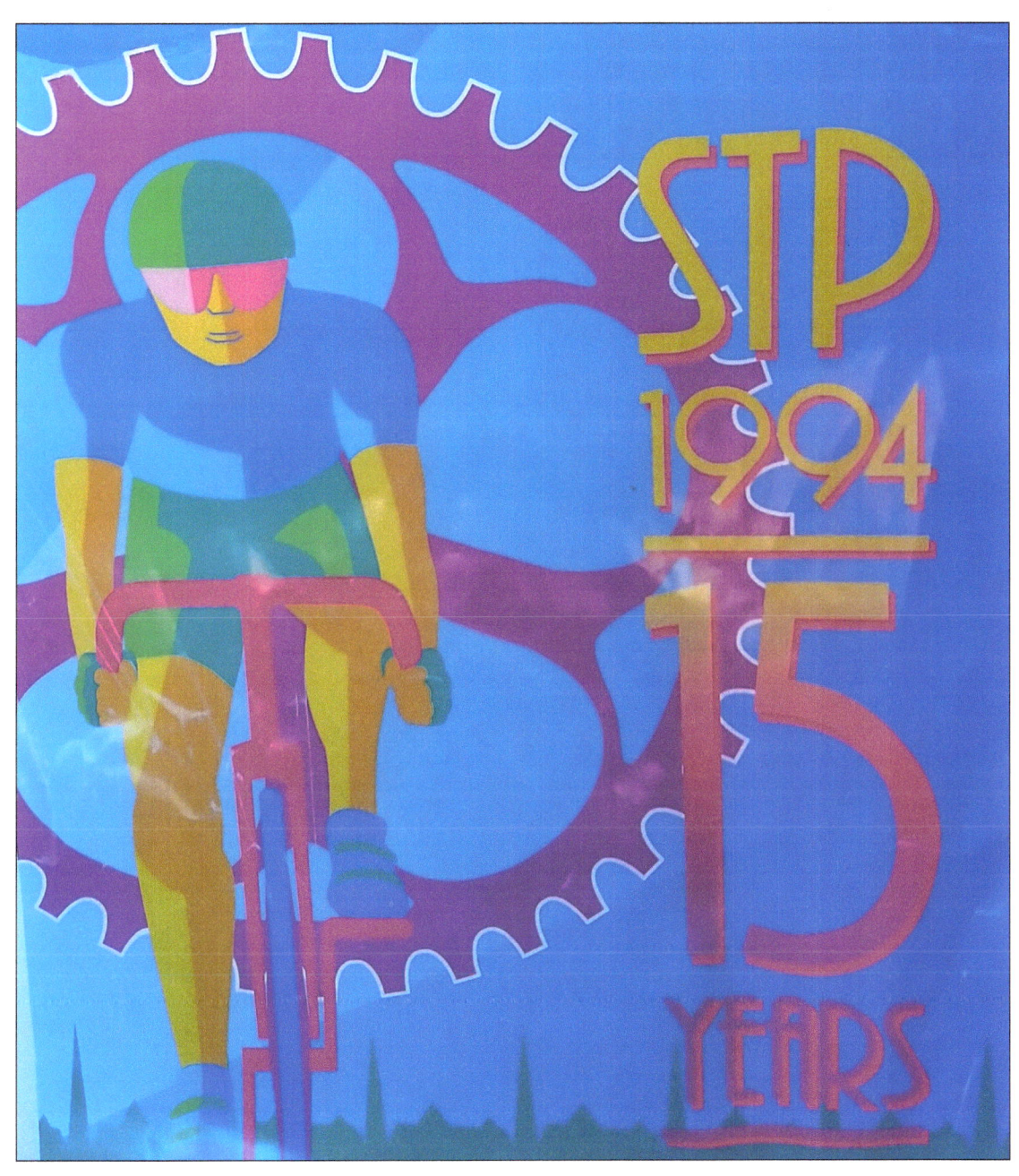

1994 *STP* 15th Anniversary Poster

*Goodness is something you do,
not something you talk about*

– Gino Bartali
Italian cycling hero and five time *'Grand Tour'* winner [26]

---

26. Gino Bartali won the *Giro d'Italia* three times and the *Tour de France* twice, before *and* after WWII.

CRASH! The Great Highway Romp and Getting 'Doored'[27] (1999)

The late 1990s was a great time for riding with my colleagues from the California Coastal Commission. I'd spent twenty years running the agency's cartography operations so other staff often saw me decked out in my helmet, riding togs and backpack, arriving or leaving work on one of my *five* bikes. Even the non cycling staff regularly stopped by my office to marvel at my two wheeled thoroughbreds. I had plenty of opportunities to ride with other Commission employees over the years and introduced many of them to some of the longer distance and larger group *century* rides that I was doing at the time.[28]

There were two younger colleagues in particular who shared my level of passion for cycling as sport. Darryl Rance and Jay Banaag both had a similar competitive nature and the three of us often met up on weekends to do serious training rides. Riding together we became friends, not just coworkers. It was some of the best training and most fun you could ever have on a bike. It was not the bliss inducing type of cycling, but nonetheless always a pleasure to ride with these two exceptional athletes.

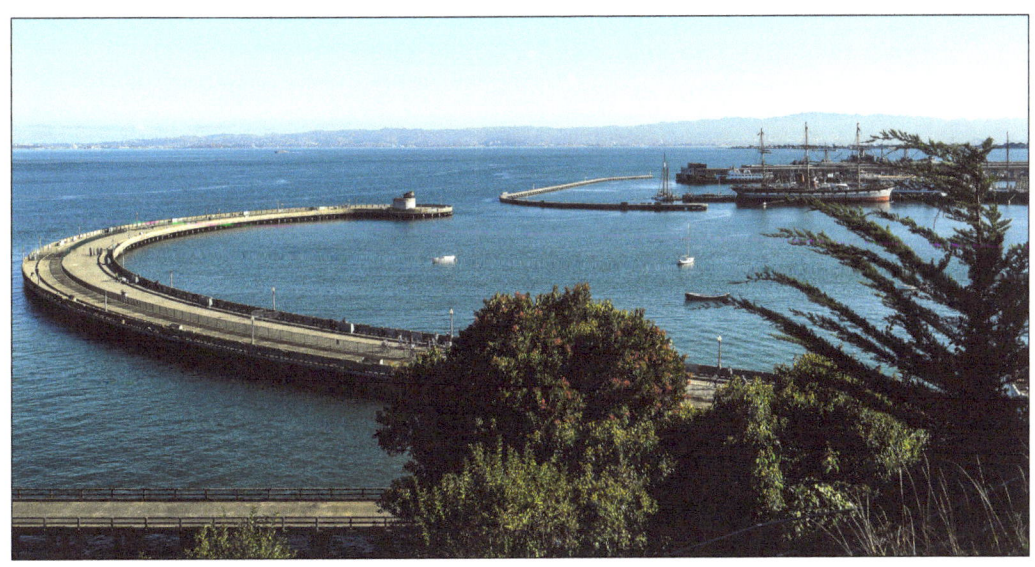

San Francisco's Aquatic Park and historic Hyde Street Pier

---

27. Getting 'doored' is the colloquial term used to describe the cycling accident that occurs when the occupant (driver) of a parked car inattentively (and illegally) opens their door into the path of an oncoming bicyclist.
28. 100 kilometer or 100 mile rides usually sponsored by a cycling club.

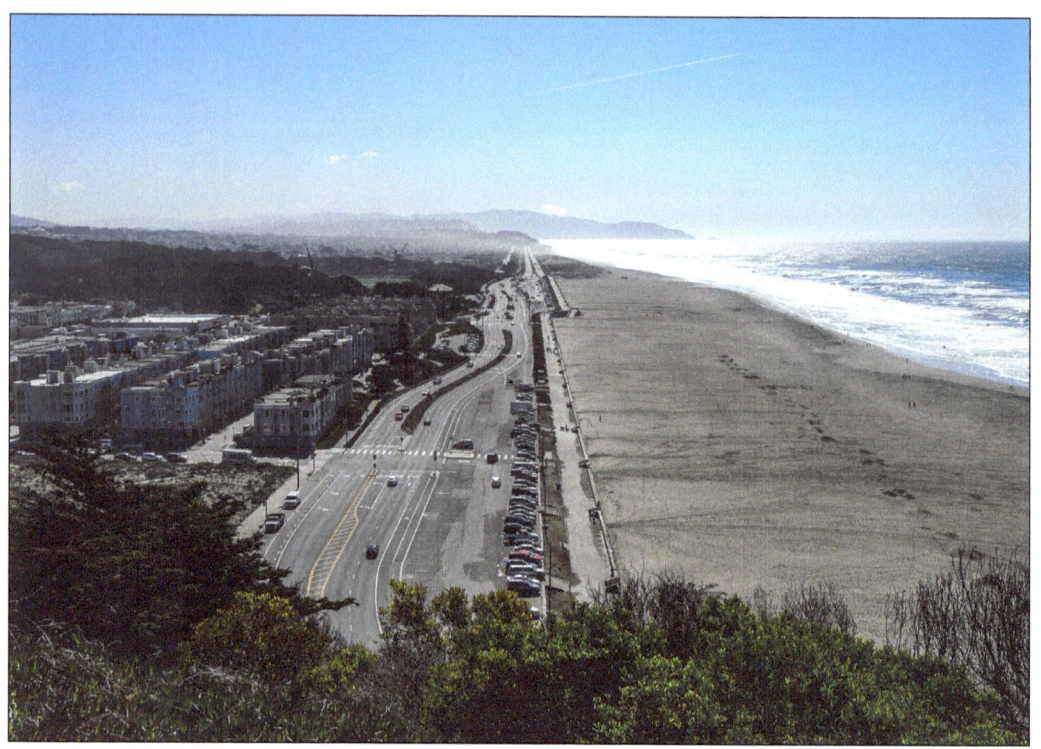

Ocean Beach and the Great Highway, San Francisco

Some of my Italian friends call me *'Il Fortunato,'* the Fortunate One, and it was certainly my good fortune to be riding with these two friends from work one Spring Saturday in 1999. A mid day sea breeze was steady – Darryl, Jay and I had decided to do 'Bayline,' a ride west following the San Francisco Bay shoreline that headed down the coast. Our plan was to stop at Lake Merced and decide whether we had time to also climb nearby San Bruno Mountain.

It was the era of narrow, high pressure tires, intended to lower a bicycle's overall rolling resistance. I was riding on a 19 mm width tire in front, and a 23 mm[29] tire on the rear, both inflated to 110 psi, or so. The popular notion was that tires less than an inch wide – pumped rock hard – would produce a rough, but faster ride. All things considered, I might have been better off riding for an hour on the cycle track in Golden Gate Park that day!

As we reached the Cliff House I remarked about the strong breeze. The sky was blue and the air was fresh. In the distance beach sand was swirling inland over our route – the Great Highway.[30] We reached the road below – just inland of the beach – and found the bike lane south of Golden Gate Park covered with a

---

29 25 millimeters equals approximately one inch
30. Occasionally this four lane, divided road must be closed for sand removal.

nearly continuous layer of sand. Riding in tire tracks of the vehicle lane was the only way for us to avoid the accumulated sand.

It was a sunny Saturday afternoon and traffic was moving at freeway speeds! With two southbound lanes car drivers could simply change lanes to maneuver around us but the ebb and flow of vehicles with the signal lights still forced us repeatedly to move to the right – out of the vehicle lane. We also had to jump a one inch gap in the pavement in order to ride briefly in the sand covered bike lane while groups of cars zoomed by.

Unfortunately, that 'one inch' gap was wider and uneven where the asphalt had been distorted by years of exposure to the elements. Night and day, sunny or grey, the salty, damp ocean air had taken a toll on the pavement, pulling apart the seams and separations in the sections of road surface.

Each of us took pulls in front as we crossed the alphabetically named streets, staying at the edge of the car lane and following a line through the thinnest film of sand in the bike lane, when necessary. The cross headwind was steady and we crouched low, rotating positions in our three man paceline. After my turn in the lead, I slotted in behind Darryl and Jay took the next pull in front. I heard cars approaching and someone's horn blaring. As I glanced back quickly, I could see a green muscle car speeding in our same southerly direction.

Santiago is the street named for the letter 'S' and the one indelibly marked in my memory. I knew 'muscle car' guy would run the light but I didn't expect him to wail on his horn as he flew by me. I flinched in response as I instinctively moved to the right and that was it – in an instant my 19 mm front tire slipped into that *wider than one inch gap* in the asphalt!

Doing an *'Endo'* is an ugly spectacle no matter what the cause. You hit something, flip the bike – back wheel up over the front wheel – and catapult off the bike. The faster you're going the harder it is to control how you hit the ground. Injuries can be serious and bikes can become trash. In this case, I launched from the bike and suffered a concussion and abrasions to my right shoulder. Somehow my *Colnago* had escaped major damage – with only scratches and rotated handlebars.

The concussion was clearly the most serious immediately outcome. I was knocked unconscious – 'out on my feet' as they say in boxing jargon – *for 45 minutes!* Luckily for me, Darryl and Jay heard metal scraping on pavement behind them and stopped immediately. To this day, I have absolutely no memory of the hour long aftermath but suffice it to say both of them acted heroically. They got me *and* my bike out of the road – telling me later that I was up and talking to them right away. Somehow they figured out that I was at least semi okay and Jay took off to get his truck while Darryl waited with me and put up with my repeated questions about what had just happened.

My direct recollection returned before Jay got back with his truck. He and Darryl wanted to take me to the hospital but I refused. Looking back now, I realize that was a mistake – partly made due to being in mild shock – but I was also being stupidly *macho* and had no clue whatsoever about concussion protocols. As far as I was concerned, I'd scraped up my shoulder and my friends had scraped *me* up. I wanted to go home, where I could check over my bike and clean up. Reluctantly, they complied.

My shoulder had a good size abrasion and was sore from the impact but that was it. My jersey had shredded at the upper arm and absorbed the tearing action of sliding. Back at home, I tried to piece together what had happened as I cleaned myself up and examined my bike. Brake lever and pedal scratches – I pondered how much worse it could have been. I'd already cracked a couple of helmets and broken my hip bicycling but this could have been 'lights out.' I called my girlfriend.

As 'fortunato' as I was that day, I wasn't so lucky with the phone call. She was upset about my crash and perhaps understandably angry that I hadn't gone to the hospital. Being scolded like a kid was absolutely *not* what I needed at that moment. I was saved 'by the bell' when my buddy Frank called to say he had arrived from Seattle. He brought me dinner and snored on my couch that night – just the right amount to wake me up from time to time, which, I learned later is proper concussion treatment protocol. It goes to show that friends can be helpful even without intending to be – or even knowing it!

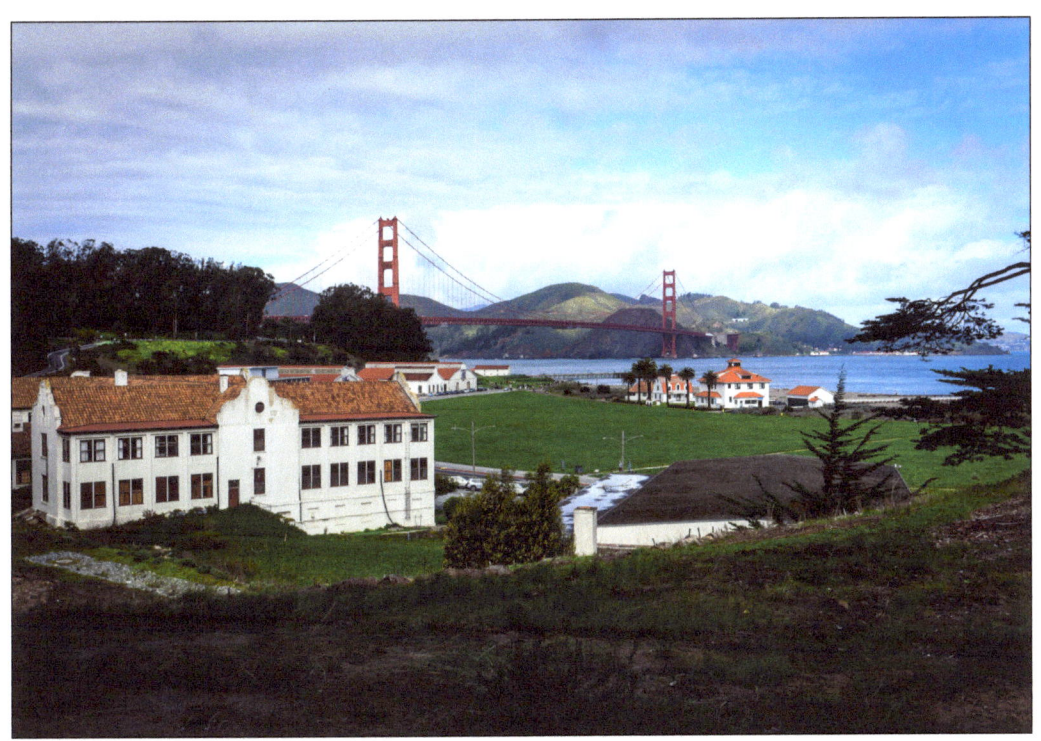

Crissy Field and the Golden Gate Bridge, Presidio of San Francisco

Fall weather is strikingly beautiful in San Francisco. The Bay Area's famous layers of advection fog thin out as atmospheric high pressure systems persist, bringing what is referred to locally as 'Indian Summer.'[31] Afternoons are warm and clear, daytime breezes are mostly light. Sunsets are amazing – September and October are two of the best months of the year for mild weather cycling in the San Francisco region.

So, there I was on a Sunday afternoon in mid September of 1999 contemplating where to take a solo ride on the bike I called 'Greenie.' This was my second *Colnago* racing bike – a newer 1990s model – a British racing green beauty with bright yellow decals. A short wheelbase 'stunner,' with straight forks, indexed shifting and dual-pivot rim brakes. *Wow!* Not only comfortable – this bike was *fast* – it handled so well on descents that I've never again even considered having a bike without straight forks. The *Campagnolo* brakes were super responsive and the action so much stronger than their *Super Record* model of a decade earlier. I loved going downhill on this bike but a great descent requires

---

31. Advection fog is a type of fog that forms when warmer, moist air flows over a colder land or water surface.

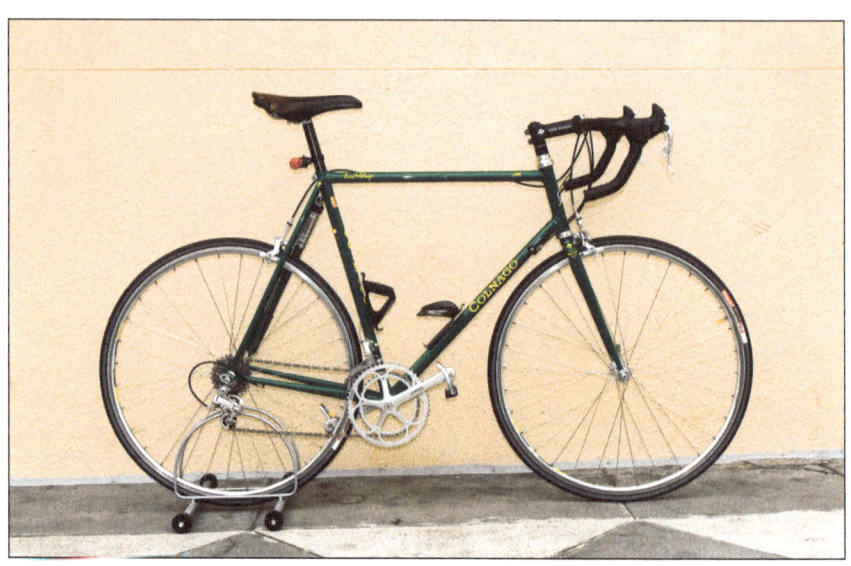

'Greenie' – aka my 1995 *Colnago Master*

a climb of some degree, so I decided to ride west along the San Francisco Bay shoreline and down the coast to Daly City, where I would climb to the top of San Bruno Mountain at an elevation of roughly 1,250 feet.

It's a great middle distance ride at roughly 45 miles, with the route profile including about 3,000 feet of climbing. Except for San Bruno Mountain, itself, the climbing sections are not that steep or sustained. It was a stunningly clear, *Indian Summer* day – I was certain the views and descent from the highest elevation on the northern San Francisco peninsula would make it worth the effort. The route profile is a classic 'bell shaped curve' – the return following a reverse of the outbound route. I rolled through the urban terrain of Daly City and climbed Guadalupe Parkway to Radio Road, then on to the 1,250 foot summit of San Bruno Mountain.[32] The views were spectacular and I thoroughly enjoyed the 'payback,' returning along the first, technical, then sinuous, two mile descent back into Daly City.

By 4 pm or so I was rolling through Fort Mason on my way back to North Beach when I chanced upon the *Day 2* headliners performing in the *San Francisco Blues Festival*. John Lee Hooker, Dr. John and several other well known greats happened to be playing their late afternoon sets in the Great Meadow. I decided to pause my ride home and enjoy the music for a while. I tucked my helmet into my backpack

---

32. The actual peak of San Bruno Mountain sits just above 1,300 feet. The summit parking area is lower.

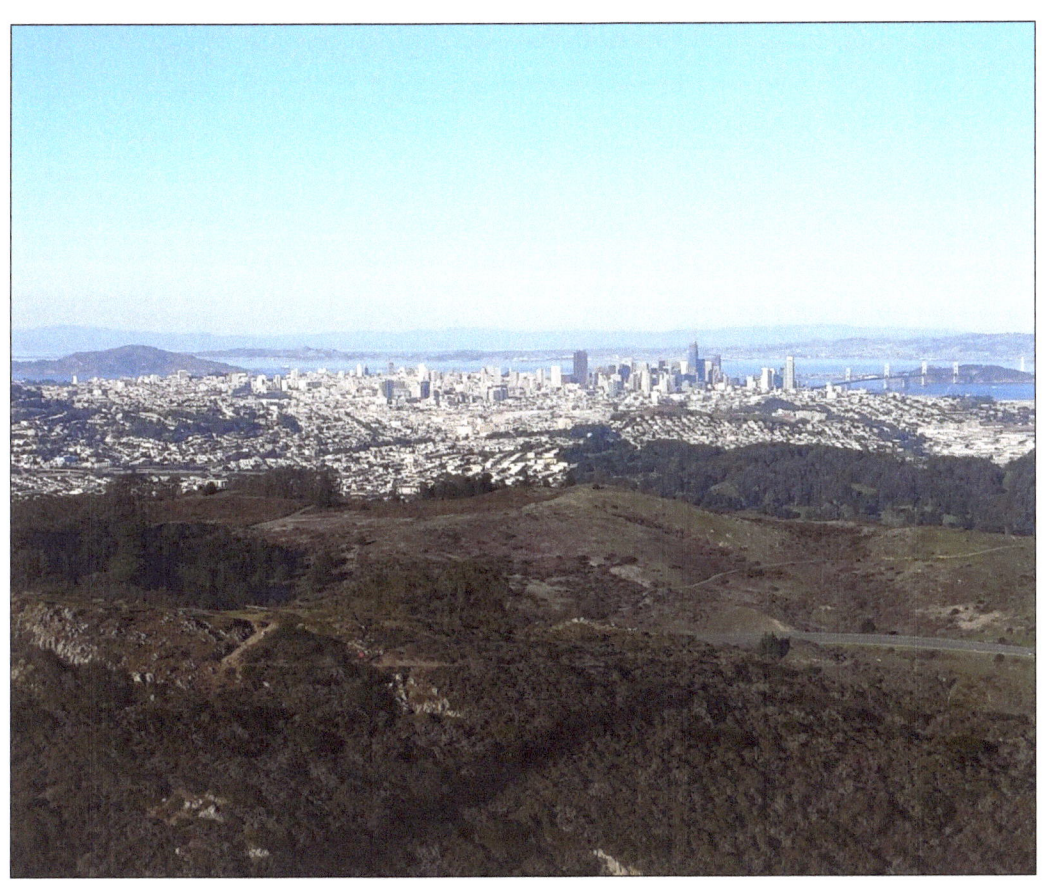

Vew north towards downtown San Francisco from San Bruno Mountain

and relaxed for an hour before riding my last mile and a half home. It was a *fantastic* show and one of John Lee Hooker's last performances.

I decided to head home at some point and I'm not sure why but I didn't put my helmet on. Maybe I rationalized that I was just fifteen minutes from home. The fact remains – I put on my backpack with the helmet still inside, unintentionally placed with its bottom against my back and the top facing out. This seemingly unimportant detail would turn out to prevent me from hitting my head five minutes later when I flew from my bike after being *doored!*

It happened in a flash – as I was riding southbound along Columbus Avenue, a divided, four lane thoroughfare. A Muni bus approached behind me and passed on the left just as the driver's door of a parked car suddenly flew open in front of me. There was no time to stop and nowhere to go! I veered as far left as possible but the bus was there. Somehow, I avoided plowing directly into the door but the car's window frame hooked my handlebars.

Accidents often seem to happen in slow motion but in an instant I was down. In a stunt-like sequence of movements, I first hit the door window frame in such a way that it abruptly stopped my forward motion. Then my rear wheel rose off the ground and my entire bike rotated, like a telescope, nearly 180 degrees – with me still on it! As gravity prevailed, the rear wheel hit the ground again and I was launched from the bike backwards, hitting the ground in a sitting position and doing what might be described as a 'reverse sit-up.'

It's difficult to visualize but I didn't hit my head! My helmet – positioned the way it was in my pack – hit the ground first and distributed the impact of landing to my back. Aside from a bleeding knuckle, I was okay. The car's driver kept apologizing and explained that he and his wife were on their way to the airport. He had forgotten something in their room at the nearby motor lodge. "Man – I don't know where you're from but this is San Francisco... you're supposed to look before getting out of your car." It was all I could say.

His wife got out of the car and began screaming when she saw blood dripping from my hand. I was holding a handkerchief but knuckle scrapes often take a while to clot. In my post accident adrenaline rush, I found her annoying and distracting. I couldn't keep myself from asking her to go back to the car while her husband and I exchanged information. I checked my bike for damage and save for a rotated stem and handlebars, there appeared to be none. A couple of new scratches on the pedals and quick release levers, no head injury... I was good to go – or so I thought. I pedaled home feeling *pissed*, but fortunate.

Two weeks later my hand had healed enough for me to resume my routine rides – now wearing a helmet regardless of where or how long I was riding. I came home from a Saturday ride and was surprised to find a fat business envelope from a law firm stuffed into my mailbox. A car rental company claiming to own the car occupied by the guy who had *doored* me was demanding that I pay over $10,000 for the damage I had 'caused' to their vehicle! I was outraged – I could have legitimately gone to the emergency room claiming neck injuries – instead, I was being subjected to a completely bogus claim.

It was time to 'play hard ball' and I told my story to a neighborhood friend, also an attorney. He recommended that I contact a well established San Francisco law firm which I promptly did. The firm of *Bianco and Bianco* promptly agreed to handle the matter and immediately, the demanding letters from lawyers ceased. Resolving the case took another three years – and a lot more time and legal work than expected – but ultimately, I received a settlement for both getting doored *and* having to respond to false claims.

I used part of that settlement to purchase a handmade, custom fit frameset, premium wheels and top components for the bike that I still ride. I also made a 'bucket list' dream come true – I financed a trip to France and saw the 2006 *Tour de France*, firsthand.

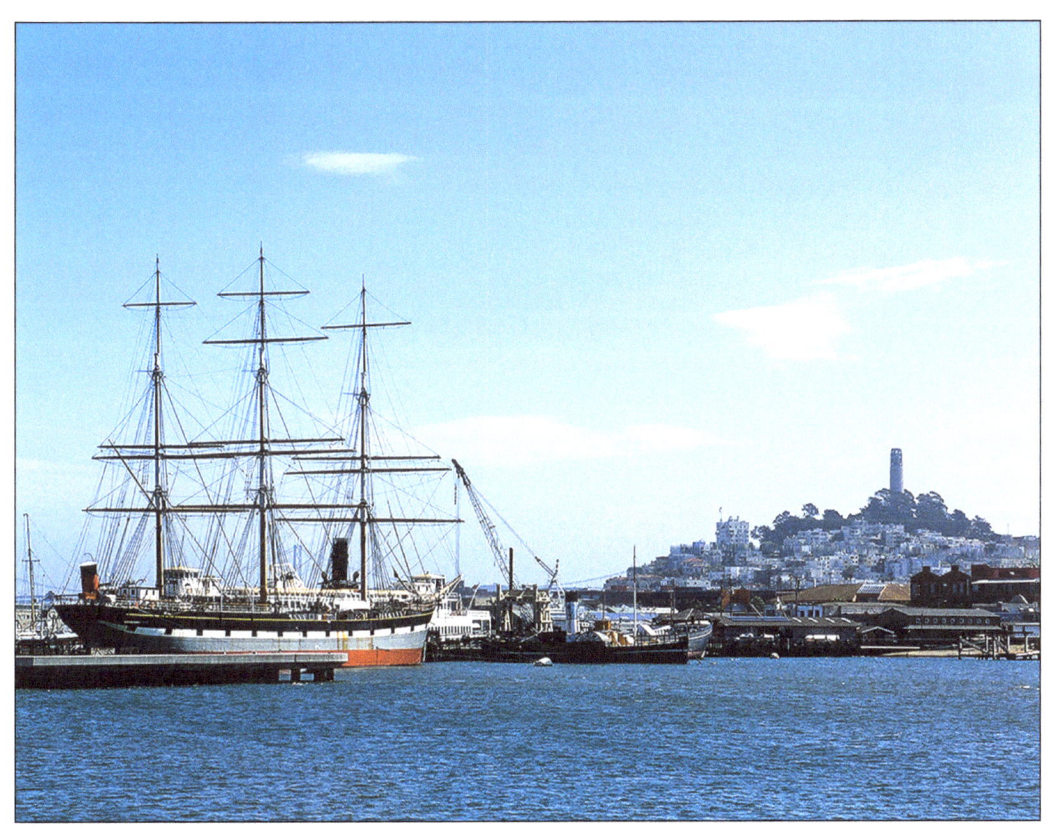

The historic sailing ship Balclutha, Telegraph Hill and Coit Tower, San Francisco

Every day there is something that reminds me why I love this sport

–BERNARD HINAULT
French cycling legend and five time winner of the *Tour de France* [33]

---

33. Bernard Hinault's *147* professional cycling victories include numerous one day Classics, Stage races and *ten* Grand Tour wins (5 *Tour de France*, 3 *Giro d'Italia* and 2 *Vuelta a España*), second only to Belgian Eddy Merckx's record of eleven. Hinault won both the *Giro d'Italia* and UCI World Championships road race in 1980. He was also a *double* Grand Tour winner in 1978, 1982 and 1985.

My Very Own *'Tour de France'* (2006)

Getting There

I first learned about professional bike racing and the world famous *Tour de France* during my teenage years. It was in the late 1960s, the era of the great Belgian champion Eddy Merckx.[34] During the years since then I often pondered actually *being* there and seeing 'The World's Greatest Bike Race.' It was something that motivated me to travel and spectate at numerous bike races all over California. I was even fortunate enough to see Olympic cycling events in Los Angeles in 1984 and the 1986 UCI[35] World Cycling Championships in Colorado. However, it wasn't until 2006 that I had the opportunity to travel in France and spend the entire month of July witnessing the *Tour de France* unfold.

To use cycling parlance and make quite a long story short, I'd been 'doored'[36] in 1999 and the ensuing legal matter took several years to be resolved but eventually I received a modest settlement. I was compensated for both getting doored *and* having to respond to false claims. I used that settlement to purchase a handmade, custom fit Mikkelsen[37] frameset, 'top shelf' wheels and components for a bike that I still ride. I had it custom painted a 'fire engine' red at D & D Cycles[38] and also made that longtime dream of mine happen – I financed a trip to France and saw the 2006 *Tour de France*.

---

34. Without question, Eddy Merckx dominated European professional cycling in the late 1960s and the 1970s. His *525* race victories include everything from numerous one-day Classics and Stage races to a record *eleven* Grand Tours. His records of 34 stage wins and *five* overall victories in the Tour de France have been equaled as of 2022 but still stand. Three time winner of the UCI World Championships road race, Merckx also set a new world record 'one hour' distance of 47.431 km (29.4 mph) in 1972 and was winner of the 'Triple Crown' (Tour de France, Giro d'Italia and World Championship victories) in 1974.
35. The UCI or *Union Cycliste Internationale*, is the world governing body for competitive cycling and oversees annual World Championship road and track racing events.
36. Getting 'doored' is the colloquial term used to describe the cycling accident that occurs when the occupant (driver) of a parked car inattentively (and illegally) opens their door into the path of an oncoming bicyclist.
37. Bernie Mikkelsen is a highly respected, master frame builder based near San Francisco in Alameda, California.
38. Master painter Rick Stefani, owner of D & D Cycles in San Lorenzo, California painted all of my racing bikes.

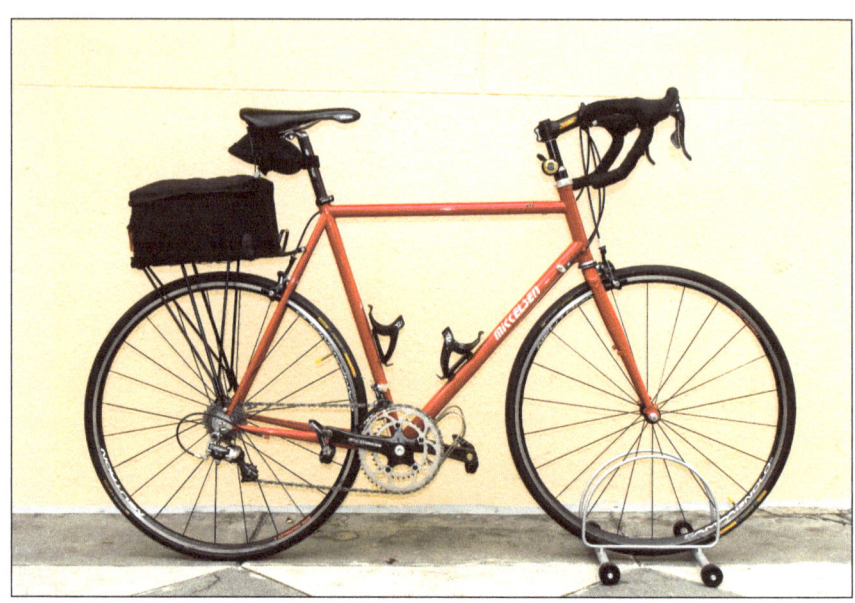

The 'Red Mikk' aka my 2006 custom *Mikkelsen*

My cycling buddy Frank and I sketched out a perfect cycling adventure – our own '*Tour de France*.' A business trip for him and a vacation for me during which we would ride our own bicycles on some of the historic *Tour de France* race routes and watch several stages[39] of the 93rd Tour in person – including the finish in Paris on the final day of the race.[40] Of course, I had no idea at the time how profoundly professional cycling would be affected by the events that took place immediately before, during and after the 2006 race. We were there to witness *Operación Puerto*[41] unfolding in the background of our trip. Titans would tumble as a large scale doping scandal and numerous ugly truths were revealed. All of the memorable fun and excitement we enjoyed on our five week sojourn took place as a monumental turning point for all of professional cycling was reached.

Having six months or so to work out a plan, Frank and I proceeded to create an ideal 28 day itinerary. We would base ourselves in Paris and travel southeast between there and Le Côte d'Azur by car – giving us the opportunity to visit, do business and bicycle in Paris and Fontainebleau, La Bourgogne, the Rhône-Alpes, La Provençe *and* the Alpes-Maritimes. I studied each region's

---

39. The 2006 Tour de France included a prologue, 20 stages and two rest days.
40. The events set in motion by revelations at the July 2006 Tour de France marked the beginning of the end of systematic 'industrial-scale' doping operations among the top teams and racers in the professional cycling peloton.
41. *Operación Puerto* is the code name for the doping investigation begun by Spanish authorities in May, 2006.

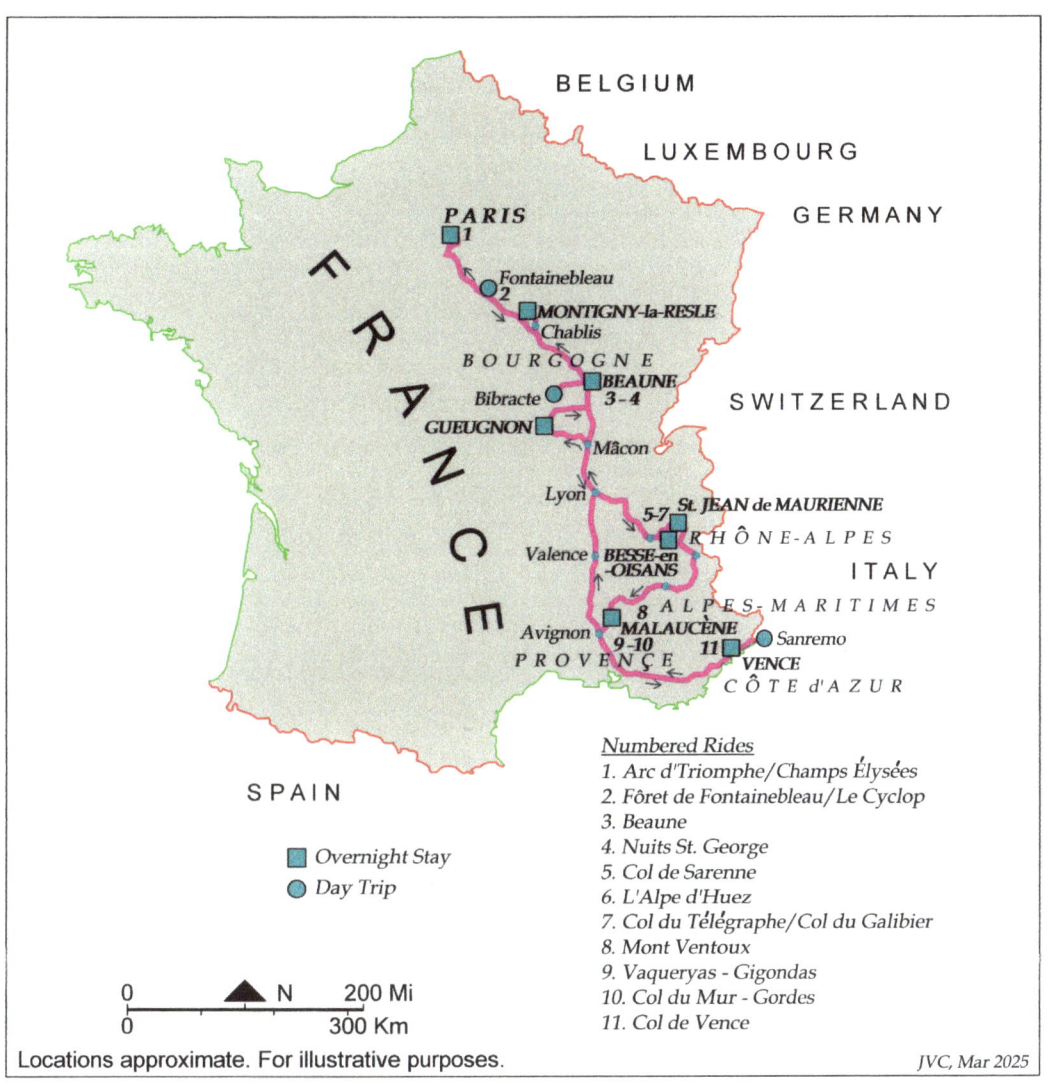

My very own 'Tour de France'

geography and mapped out rides and sightseeing trips. As one might imagine, exceptional wine and great food were also on the agenda. In the end, all went flawlessly and we had a great time – *sans incident!*

I left San Francisco on Tuesday, June 27th *en route* nonstop to Paris on Air France. Once in the air I settled into my aisle seat and ordered champagne – a tasty, French brut. My dinner – a salmon fillet and vegetables – was fit for first class and presaged the many exceptional meals I would enjoy throughout July. Thunderstorms and crying babies made it a long sleepless night but I read *VeloNews*,[42] chatted with an Italian couple returning home from their California vacation, watched a bad movie and dozed a bit.

---

42. A popular printed bicycling periodical of the day that routinely covered professional racing in Europe. VeloNews has been in publication since March 1972.

As we approached French airspace passengers became active and more talkative. The morning sky was hazy but the countryside north of Paris looked green and beckoning from above. The banter increased as the plane descended and I noticed how much I enjoyed hearing people speak French. A fair number of words sounded familiar but I couldn't really understand many phrases. I heard an accent on the last syllable of words. I was curious and looked forward to being in a place where I would have to attempt communicating in another language.

The flight distance was about 5,600 miles, the travel time – roughly 11 hours. All in all, getting there went smoothly. Flying directly to Paris had been the right choice. I resolved to record my experiences during this 'once in a lifetime' trip in a daily journal that became the basis for the story presented here nineteen years later.

I transcribed my journal upon returning to San Francisco and ended up with a thirty page document! Later on, as I considered creating this *cycling geographer's* story, I decided to focus on people, places, rides and races… and of course, food and drink! I've attempted to leave out the banal, however, there are no doubt many details that remain, perhaps of more interest to geographers, serious cyclists or food connoisseurs.

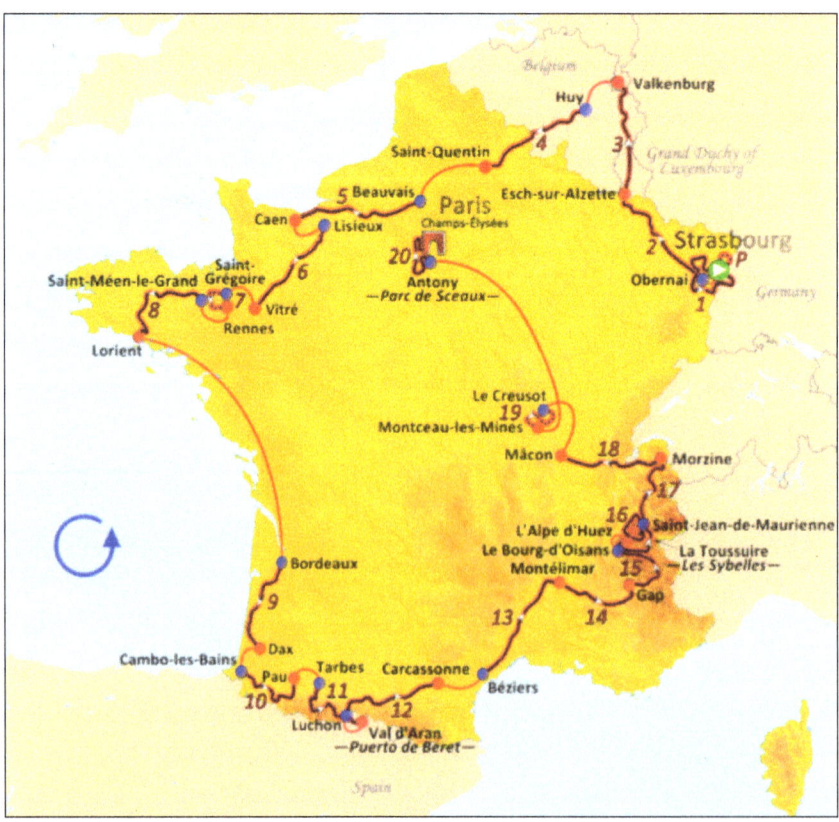

Route of the 2006 Tour de France

Paris, Fontainebleau and Le Cyclop

After arriving at Charles de Gaulle airport mid day Wednesday I met my limo driver Stephane and headed into Paris through slow moving traffic. There was Frank looking down from a second floor balcony as I reached Rue de Folie Mericourt in the neighborhood known as L'République. The apartment was perfect – a nice, modern studio – entirely adequate for the two of us. Bikes on the balcony, bike bags under the bed and luggage in the closet and corners... It was to make a great 'base camp,' situated at the juncture of the 3rd, 10th and 11th arrondissements[43] near the Canal Saint-Martin. The location was within walking distance of the River Seine, close to cafes and anything we needed.

Early the next day Frank and I strolled to what became our regular cafe each morning while in Paris, *La Grissette. Petit déjuener*[44] – a fresh baguette and coffee – was served up within moments. The people watching was excellent and the early morning temperature was 68°F (20°C) – under clear summer skies.

The morning commute was amazing to witness from *La Grisette*. The streets were filled with bicycles. Without a doubt, thousands of bicyclists are on the streets in Paris every day! Bike lanes on the main thoroughfares are physically separated from

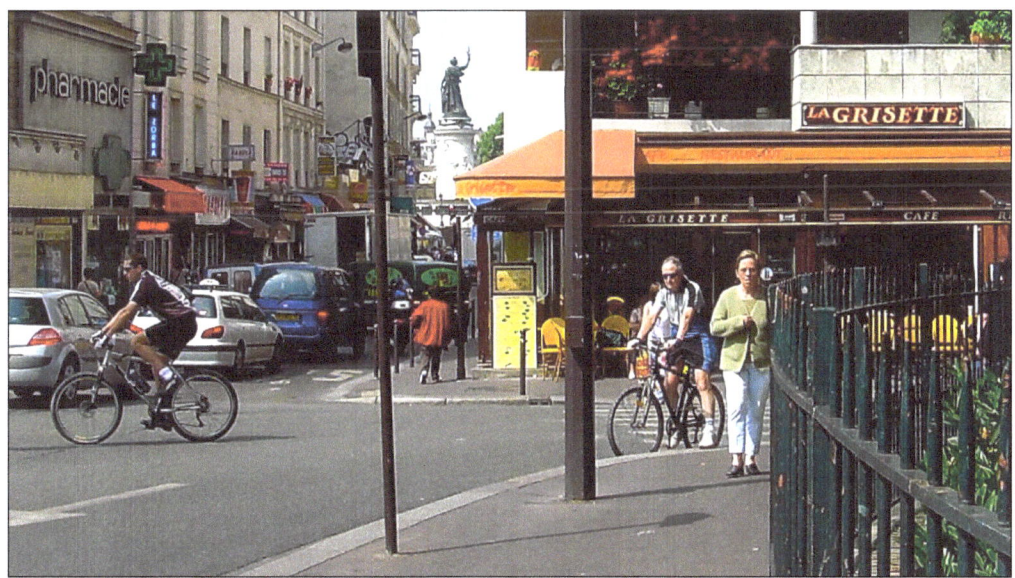

La Grissette, near the Canal Saint-Martin in L'République, Paris

---

43. The Paris arrondissements are the City's urban administrative districts.
44. Breakfast

the auto traffic lanes. Of course, there are lots of scooters and motorcycles – pedestrians, too. A blur of ruddy faced men and stylish women streamed by – so many riding bikes. I found myself focused on the women passing by looking fit and fashionable, whether on two wheels or not.[45]

That afternoon Frank and I suited up and went for our first bike ride in France – along the River Seine and through the heart of Paris! We followed the Canal Saint-Martin to the Seine, crossed at Pont du Austerlitz and then rode along the quais [46] on the left bank of the River, past the mint, the École des Beaux Arts, the Musee d'Orsay, the National Assembly and the Esplanade des Invalides, to the Eiffel Tower. Wow! We were both excited to see the famous route of the Tour's grand finale and rode on to the Arc d'Triomphe, the Champs Élysées, and the Place de la Concorde.

It was approaching six pm and slow going on the Champs Élysées. We had taken our time enjoying the sights and it became clear that the evening commute had begun. The 'flat' cobbles were not so flat or much fun as we maneuvered our bikes through the sluggish traffic. But what a great cycling city, regardless – the *Île de la Cité* felt intensely urban yet beautiful, green and exhilarating! Hundreds of people were out relaxing in the early evening sun along the Canal Saint-Martin, enjoying simple picnics and wine, playing music, singing, dancing – even juggling. Couples, groups of 'twenty somethings' and older folks – all enjoying themselves outside. The early July Paris weather felt comfortable and inviting. It seemed there could be no reason for remaining indoors.

After several days of exploring L'République we began preparing for our month long journey southeast to and from Le Côte d'Azur. Early Friday morning we picked up a Peugeot sedan at the Gare du Nord.[47] As one might expect, driving is complicated in Paris but Frank managed admirably – weaving in and out of the

---

45. My favorite had to be a young woman who cruised by, looking like the actress Natalie Wood in a flared skirt, flat shoes, scarf and dark glasses, holding a cell phone in one hand and a cigarette and the handlebars in the other - nonchalant on her 'step-through' style bike - completely in control while her little white terrier rode up front in a wicker basket.
46. Quais are the riverfront walkways along the River Seine in central Paris.
47. The Gare du Nord, opened in 1864, is the magnificent Paris train station on the Rue de Maubridge in the 10th Arrondissement. It is the busiest of all of the City's railroad hubs and currently undergoing remodeling in anticipation of the 2024 Olympic Games to be held in and around Paris.

lanes – speeding along while inches from other cars and trucks on the way back to our neighborhood. Like magic, we arrived to find an empty parking place directly in front of the apartment! There was now time for croissants and coffee before we loaded the bikes and drove 50 kilometers (31 miles) southeast to Fontainebleau, where we intended to stage a flat ride through the National Forest.[48]

I had mapped a route that would take us through the Forêt de Fontainebleau, a 250 square kilometer remnant of ancient forest and former royal hunting grounds.[49] We would also pass through the village of Barbizon on the way to our destination near Milly-la-Forêt: *Le Cyclop*, a gigantic mirror-covered outdoor sculpture consisting of the head of the one eyed creature emerging directly from the ground.[50] It was one of the more unusual things I'd read about in my planning and the idea of seeing it had intrigued me. Our sojourn became the first of nearly a dozen memorable rides that we would complete while in France.

We arrived at Fontainebleau in the early afternoon and parked near the famed medieval 16th century renaissance Château de Fontainebleau.[51] Though officially designated an important architectural and historic site during the early 20th century, Frank and I saw it in a surprisingly 'rough' condition. What I had assumed would be considered a national treasure was in disrepair, looking neglected with its peeling paint, broken window glass and damaged roof tiles. I was pleased to eventually learn that various extensive restoration projects have been undertaken since 2006.

---

48 One mile equals 1.61 kilometers. One kilometer equals .62 miles.
49. Under Napoleon III, the *Forêt de Fontainebleau* became the world's first nature preserve in 1861.
50. *Le Cyclop* is a 75 foot high cyclop head constructed by Swiss artist Jean Tinguely, French artist Niki de Saint Phalle and others from 350 tons of industrial debris, during the period of 1969-91. Inspired by the Dada, Nouveau Réalisme, Kinectic Art and Art Brut movements, the sculpture was opened to the public in 1994.
51. The Château is a United Nations Educational Scientific and Cultural Organization (UNESCO) World Heritage Site. Several dozen French Kings, Napoleons I and III, and numerous other modern royalty and world leaders spent important time there during the past *500* years.

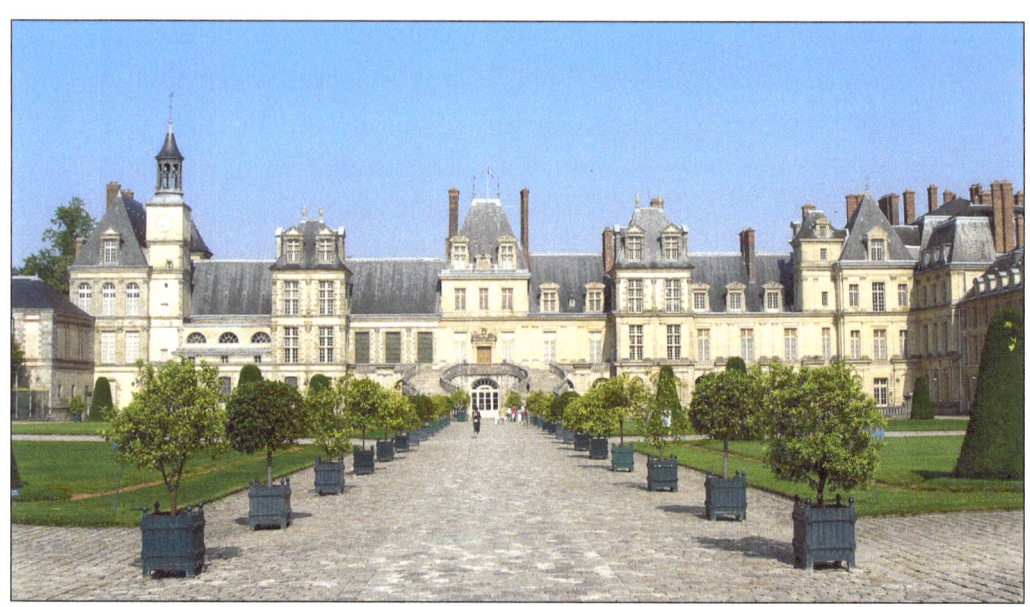

Château de Fontainebleau

We began our ride through town, making our way into the National Forest. The two lane road was in excellent shape with no traffic in sight. It was mid day and already getting hot. The mixed oak and pine canopy provided some shade but we could already smell oils and sap from the trees vaporizing in the heat. I began feeling the tingle of perspiration evaporating from my neck and forearms.

Since the forest road was closed to through traffic there were absolutely *no* motor vehicles. No other cyclists either – we had the road entirely to ourselves! All we heard was the muffled sounds of warblers and woodpeckers. Our route took us through an area of massive sandstone boulders where we passed a small group of campers but otherwise we were alone. Visualize two fit riders rolling along carefree and quickly on a flat, sinuous, well paved and gated National Forest road for *20* kilometers! I soon sensed that bicycling induced, blissful feeling coming on. Frank and I didn't talk much and had no need to speak. Only the quiet whirring sounds of our bicycles accompanied the chorus of tapping, repeating bird calls and buzzing sounds coming from the woods.

We left the forest temporarily and stopped in Barbizon to get our bearings. There, we met the first of several pleasant and interesting cultured women encountered throughout our trip. A friendly faced gardener stood outside the Museum of Barbizon Painters watering flowers as we stopped to ask directions. Realizing that we didn't speak French he offered to ask the museum director to assist us. No sooner had he entered the building when an attractive middle aged woman instantly emerged. I couldn't help but notice her long dark hair drawn to the side and pastel green, flared knee-length skirt. Appearing very urbane but with a 'rural grace,' she looked naturally stylish and sophisticated but equally capable of handling the mundane.

We were lucky. The lovely *Marie* spoke English confidently and gave us clear directions while also explaining that she had studied the language for years because she felt that English allowed one a greater opportunity to write more expressively. With her enthusiasm and emotive accent she could only further affirm what I had already suspected – it's a myth that French people, in general, dislike or dismiss Americans or English speakers en masse – so far, the truth seemed far from it.

With our courteously-provided instructions we continued through Barbizon, a quaint village with that distinct feel of a hamlet that became an artist community. Many houses and buildings were stone. We had emerged from the forest onto flat roads with pastoral views of the surrounding farms and rural countryside. I imagined that these bucolic landscapes must have been painted during the 19th century by Camille Corot, Théodore Rousseau, Francois Millet and other artists who became known as the Barbizon Painters.[52] The horizon shimmered and the heat was palpable. There was a golden late afternoon light that permeated the entire scene. It looked and felt timeless.

We entered the Forêt de Trois Pignons (Three Pines) and I started wondering how and why *Le Cyclop* had come to be located *here*. Even more puzzling was why, once we had arrived at the sculpture, the attendant refused to let us in! I was annoyed but it seemed to be just before an early closing time – he clearly wanted to lock up. Despite our best attempts to assure him we would quickly take photos and leave, his attitude remained stern and authoritarian... access for visitors would not be permitted.

---

52. The 'Barbizon School' painters were pioneering plein-air artists who visited or lived there and developed a distinct style of naturalism and realism using the area's landscapes as independent subjects for their work. Their movement rejected the rigid idealized landscape depictions of the Romantic style and influenced later works of Impressionist painters such as Monet and Renoir, who also came to Barbizon and the Forêt de Fontainebleau.

I managed to traipse around the perimeter fence enclosing *Le Cyclop* looking for a hole or some separation where I could take a picture. After finding what I wanted I did my best to get a shot of the one eyed man of the hour. Frank helped me clean the dirt clods now stuck in the cleats of my cycling shoes and we decided to look for something cold to drink in the nearby village of Milly-la-Forêt before heading back.

Milly-la-Forêt was another picturesque village – with a church, château and block long covered market place. The real surprise was the *Kronenbourg!*[53] Who would have thought? Ice-cold, 'industrial' French beer at the village tavern – *Le Bacchus*. It was perfect hydration for us and we were soon chatting with some locals who spoke a bit of English and even kept an eye on our bikes through the windows while we enjoyed our beers at the tiny bar. We did our best to explain why we were there but it seemed as though not many touring American bicyclists were often seen in those parts, at least not in bars wearing their cycling 'togs.[54] It was a very special place and a perfect counterpoint to our experience at the nearby sculpture. One other thing became clear... the local 'barflies' had previous knowledge that the fellow at *Le Cyclop* could be a jerk!

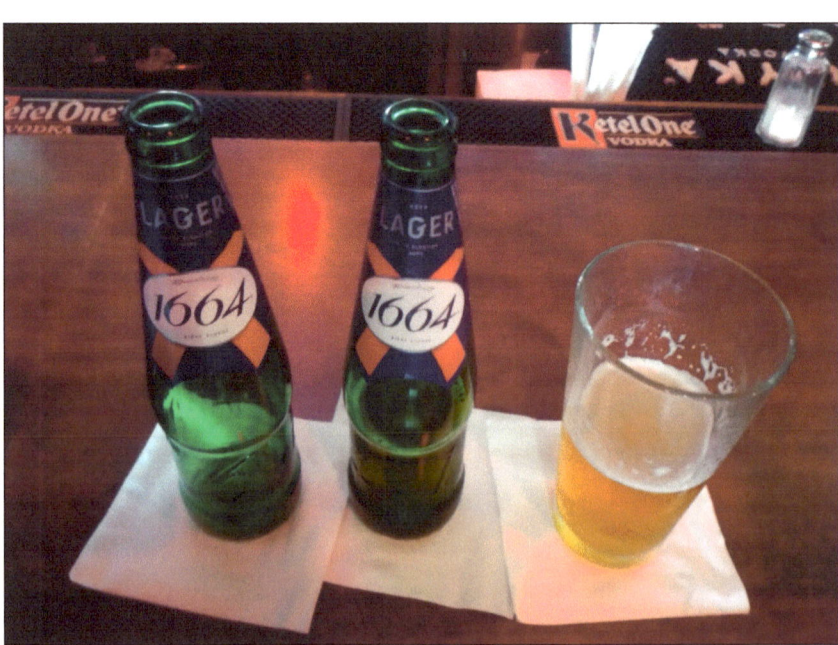

Kronenbourg 1664, French industrial lager beer

---

53. *Kronenbourg '1664'* is a 5.5% golden lager beer found throughout France.
54. Riding shoes and apparel.

Frank and I split a third refreshing Kronenbourg and then headed out into the 90°F (32°C) heat to continue our ride towards the National Forest. We were soon enveloped in the shade of late afternoon and it felt a few degrees cooler. The leafy canopy was quite high and filtered sunlight reflected on the giant boulders. I imagined a time when French monarchs and their mignons travelled through this very forest while hunting. Standing like sentinels, the mature pine trees had trunks wide enough to provide natural cover. We continued on and met the smoke and smells of campfires ahead. The chattering voices of boys and men began to overwhelm the sounds of the forest and the rolling noises of our bicycles.

Our return route took us directly through the forest and we were soon at the car in Fontainebleau. All things considered the afternoon had been great fun – a perfectly enjoyable ride. Despite the afternoon heat and slight disappointment at not having *fully* accomplished our objective, neither of us had any mechanical problems or flat tires, we'd met several interesting nice people and traversed some remarkable landscapes and natural scenery. We had experienced *two* amazing rides through the *Forêt de Fontainebleau*! All was good – it didn't matter that we had missed *Le Cyclop* 'up close.'

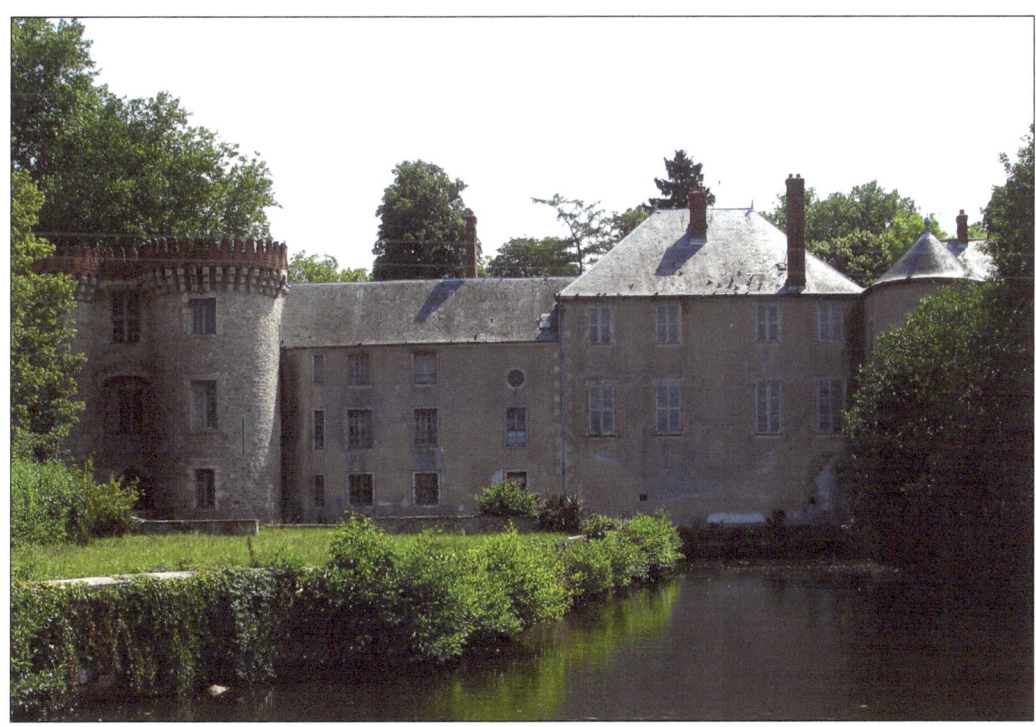

Château, Milly-la-Forêt

We strolled around the village center in Fontainebleau and stopped for a light dinner before returning to Paris. As I enjoyed my *salade niçoise* and *petite crus* chablis I couldn't help reflecting further on the ride. Frank agreed – what we had done all day was 'roll with it' and one thing after another had worked out for the best. Something I've known now for decades was affirmed – *Under the best circumstances the experience of cycling is more about the ride than the destination.*

Back in Paris our good fortune with car parking continued. We arrived in L'République to find the same previous space vacant, directly in front of our apartment – as if waiting for us! After unloading the car I went out to buy a copy of *L'Equipe*[55] and quickly figured out that something serious was going on with the Tour… the race prologue was scheduled to take place the following day but a Spanish doping investigation,[56] underway since May, had just publicly implicated 58 *Tour de France* racers! Earlier that day the 21 Team Directors had voted unanimously to remove nine riders from the event. The bad news may have been in French but its message was clear – three top contenders would *not* be allowed to start the next day in Strasbourg![57]

---

55. *L'Equipe* is a premier sports newspaper in France that provides extensive coverage of professional cycling.
56. *Operación Puerto* is the code name for the investigation by Spanish authorities into a sophisticated illegal doping program run by Spanish doctor Eufemiano Fuentes and others, including team directors. Many riders were eventually cleared while others retired or admitted their involvement and received suspensions.
57. Four racers, German Jan Ullrich, Spanish-Columbian Óscar Sevilla, Spaniard Francisco Mancebo and Italian Ivan Basso, were suspended and disqualified from the race.

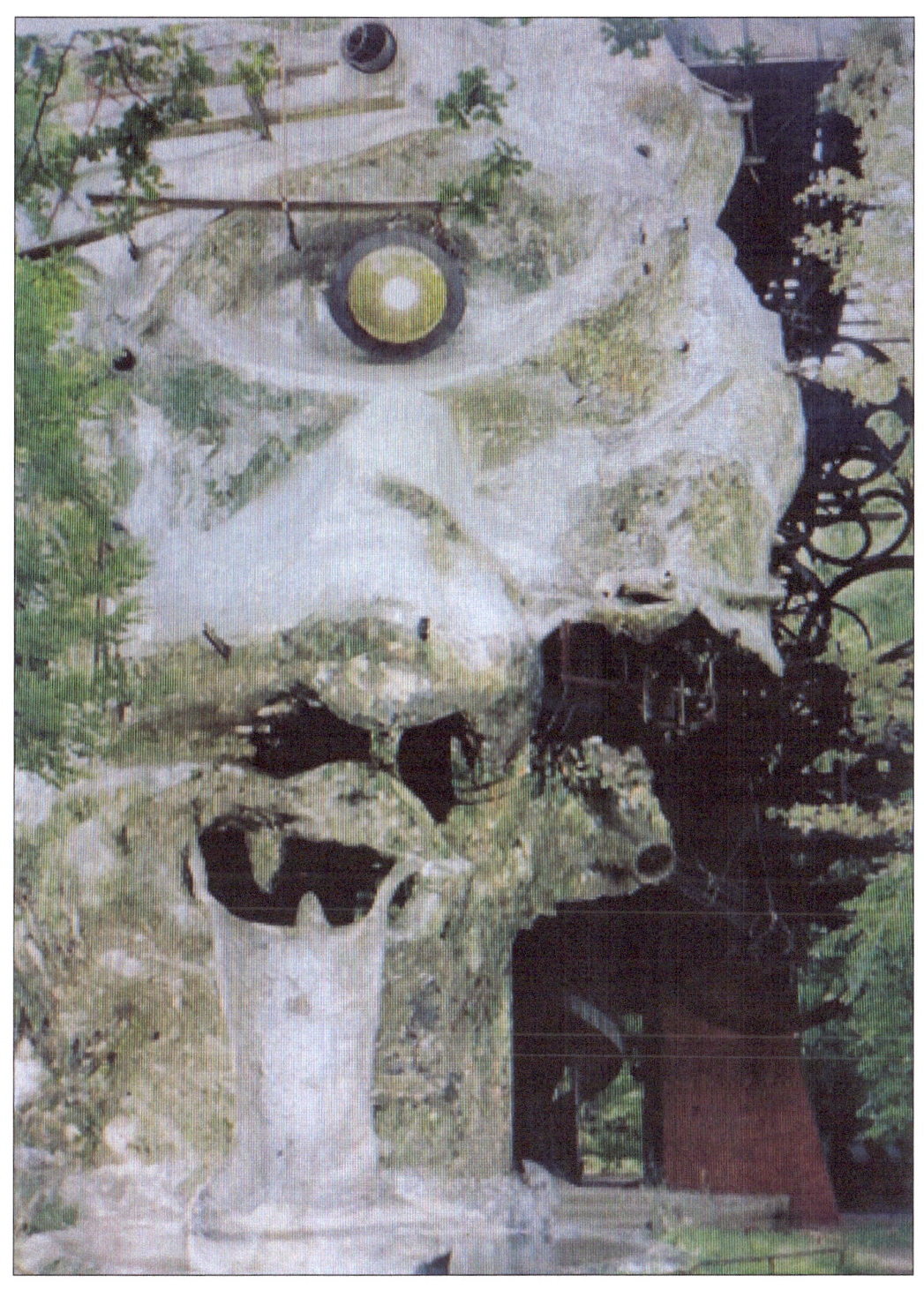

Le Cyclop is a 75 foot high cyclop head constructed from 350 tons of industrial debris

La Bourgogne

Saturday, July 1st we left Paris and headed for Montigny-la-Resle in the wine country – the Côte-d'Or,[58] where we arrived at *La Val du Chapelain* and met our hosts Pascale and Nicole Fraure. Their beautifully restored manor house was surrounded by the extensive vineyards and woodlands found in this region. It would be a short stay but a *'Five Star'* experience in a pleasant and relaxing setting that immediately reminded me of the Napa and Sonoma Valley wine country in northern California. There were countless songbirds!

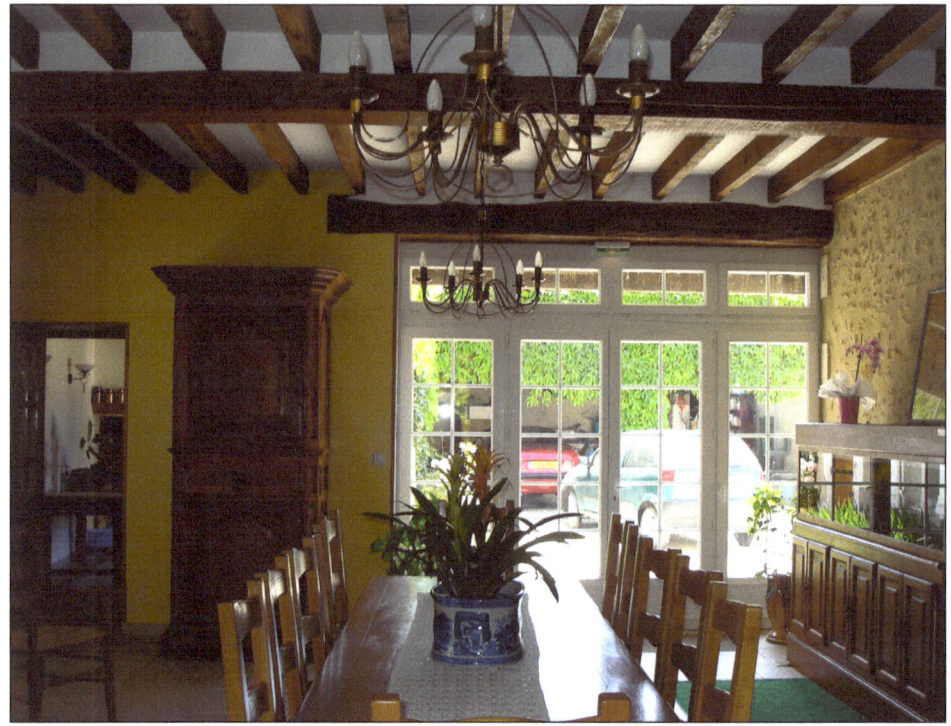

La Val du Chapelain, Montigny-la-Resle

That afternoon Frank and I went to taste our first fine wines from the region, produced by Domaine Vrignaud, a family run operation ongoing in the same location for *300 years!* We toured their newly constructed facility with Guillaume Vrignaud and his associate, Yvan Bevancof, who explained their complex modern winemaking process. Afterwards we tasted their *petit chablis, chablis, chablis premier cru* and *chablis grand cru*. There we stood in a cave nearly 400 years old, drinking 2003 (an excellent year for wine from this region) chablis grand cru produced from the fruit of 50 year old vines!

---

58. The Côte-d'Or (Golden Slope) is a department in Northeastern France famous for its fine wine. The southeast-facing slopes of the Cote d'Or limestone escarpment here are the location of many important and unique Burgundian vineyards producing pinot noir and chardonnay grapes. A UNESCO site since 2015.

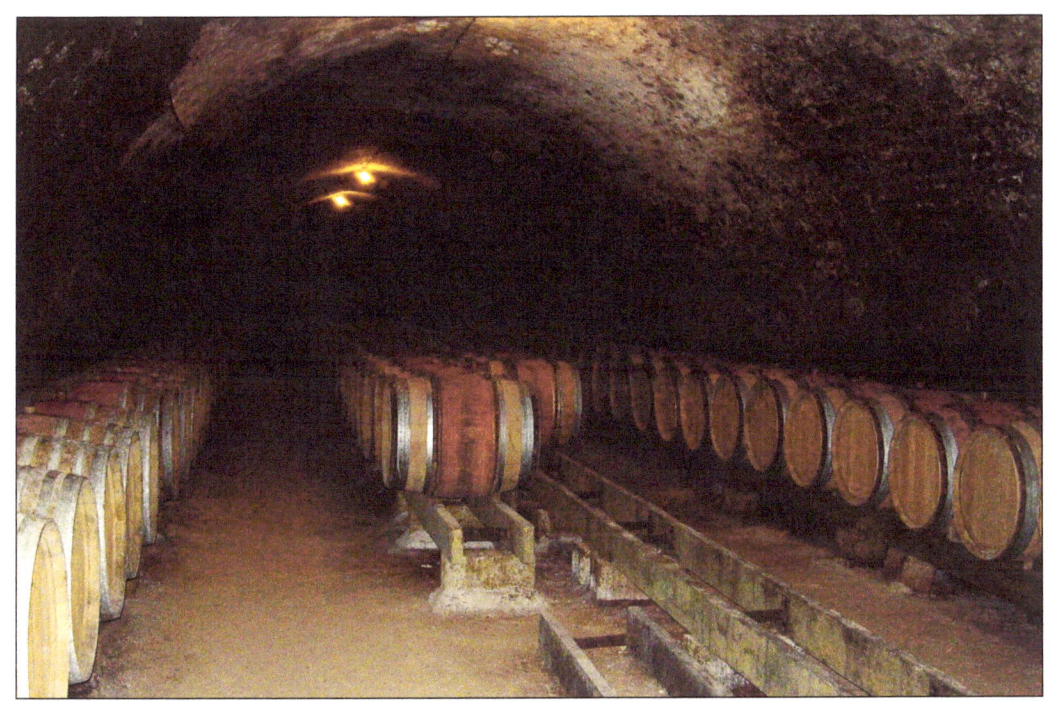

400 year old limestone cave, Domaine Vrignaud

Later on Yvan and Guillaume took us into nearby Chablis to eat and watch the World Cup *futbol* match between France and Brazil. The Chablis Bar was also a fine restaurant and we were treated to escargot and salad before an entrée of perch fillets with rice, potato *and* vegetables was served. Wow! The tomato based sauce gracing our fish was something special, as was the salad, which included not only greens but ham, andouille sausage and a dish of eggs in a red wine sauce. Guillaume chose excellent wines to accompany our meal. Everything was superb and France prevailed in the world cup competition... advancing to contest Portugal in the semi final.

After returning to La Val du Chapelain Pascale informed us that Norwegian Thor Hushovd had won the *Tour de France* prologue in Strasbourg, completing the pan flat 7.1 km time trial in eight minutes, 17 seconds, an average speed of almost 51.5 km per hour. He would be the first to wear the 2006 leader's jersey, the *maillot jeaune*.[59] Of course, the unfolding doping scandal and resultant disqualifications were also front page news. Accusations and denials of involvement and any wrongdoing were flying!

---

59. The *maillot jeaune*, or yellow jersey, is worn by the leader in the Tour's General Classification (GC).

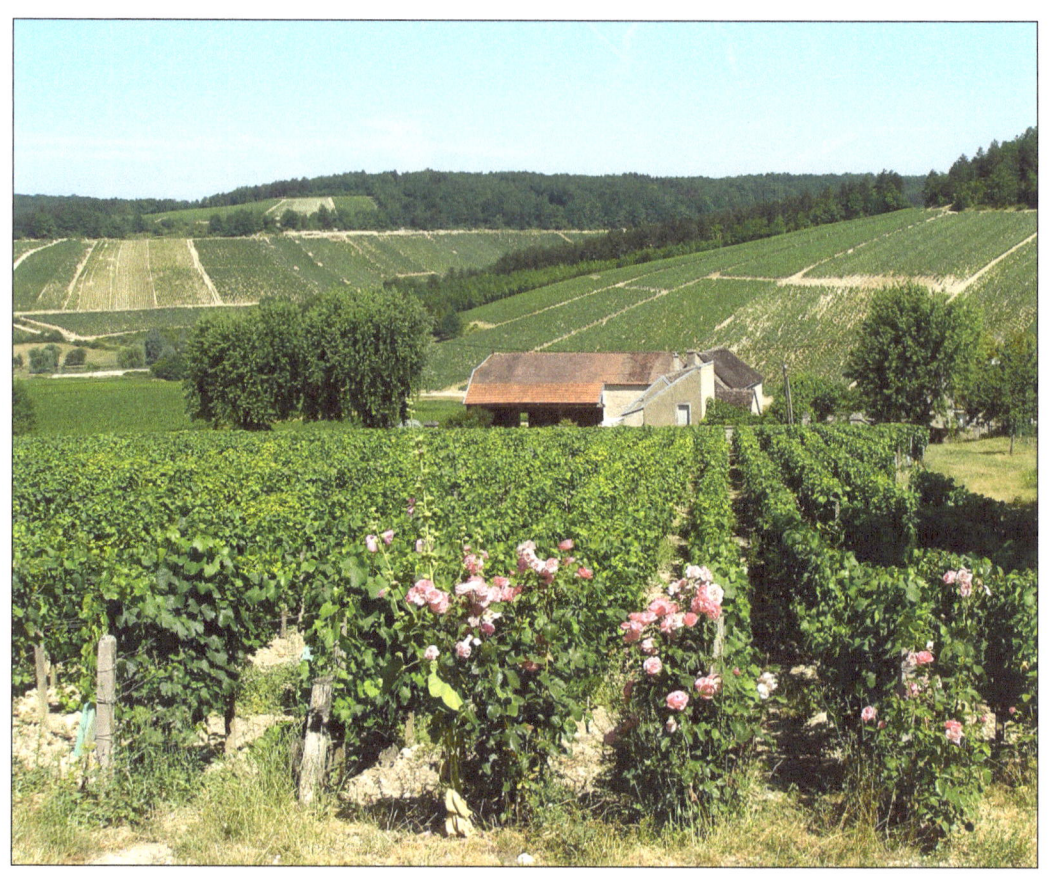

Domaine Phillipon, Chablis

Sunday morning arrived and everything looked, smelled and felt like *wine country.* We planned to travel on to Beaune but before leaving Montigny-la-Resle we stopped to visit the domaine of Andre Phillipon, a small-volume producer of *chablis,* where we tasted his excellent *chablis premier cru* and *chablis grand cru.* Spending an hour or so in his cave and barrel room made the late morning extraordinary. Besides providing respite from the rising outside temperature, the air in the cave was saturated with alcohol and the intense aromas of his wine. The high ceiling kept it feeling cool and mellow – a very relaxing space. I could feel myself ingesting alcohol simply by breathing. Through the open door Andre Phillipon's vineyards and estate looked like a perfect subject for a Barbizon style painting – the vibrant deep green and golden yellow landscape stretched out below a cloudless blue sky. Sunlight glimmered below the horizon on the whitewashed village of nearby Chablis.

We drove on to Savigny-lès-Beaune via minor highways and arrived mid afternoon. After settling into our lodgings at *Lud'Hôtel* we went into Beaune to eat and explore. We found the *Caffé Batard* and tried our first 'French' pizza and *biere pression*.[60] It was quickly becoming clear – the French don't compromise when it comes to *any* food – even simple dishes like pizza are prepared with fresh ingredients and presented with flair. The pies were typically thin crust – with no chicken, pineapple or gobs of cheese – very unlike 'American' pizza. In Beaune I understood why we'd already seen so many 'French' pizza places – in the United States it would be considered *health* food!

Back at the hotel I saw the news that Frenchman Jimmy Casper had won the Tour's mostly flat 185 km Stage 1 in four hours, 10 minutes. Top USA pro George Hincapie had taken the GC leader's *maillot jeaune* from Thor Hushovd, who was injured in a bizarre accident caused by a spectator waving a stiff cardboard sign over the barriers along the route of the race's finishing sprint! He suffered lacerations to his upper arm but received stitches immediately and was fortunately able to continue in the Tour.

The next morning Frank and I visited nearby San Romain and the *Tonnellerie François Frères*,[61] where we enjoyed a remarkable tour of the cooperage. We were shown the *entire* process of wine barrel making from the splitting, cutting and seasoning of the oak wood (sourced only from a particular region in northern France) to the milling of the staves and end pieces, band fabrication, 'toasting' of the inside surface, assembly, testing and branding of the final product. *François Frères* manufactures 161 custom ordered barrels a day, each one considered among the finest in the world.[62]

Afterwards, we returned to Savigny and suited up for an afternoon ride. Following the departmental[63] road for an hour or so north we climbed gradually towards the village of Anthueil. As in Chablis, the 'wine country' landscape around Beaune looked

---

60. Draft beer.
61. *Tonnellerie* is translated to English as *cooperage,* a facility in which casks and barrels are manufactured.
62. A family business in operation for over a century, *François Frères* is a modern industrial cooperage, however, the master carpenters and artisans are trained to use traditional hand tools as well as their automated equipment. Frank and I were also given a tour of the hand tool storeroom, which was akin to a carpenter's museum!
63. *Departments* in France might be compared to counties in the United States.

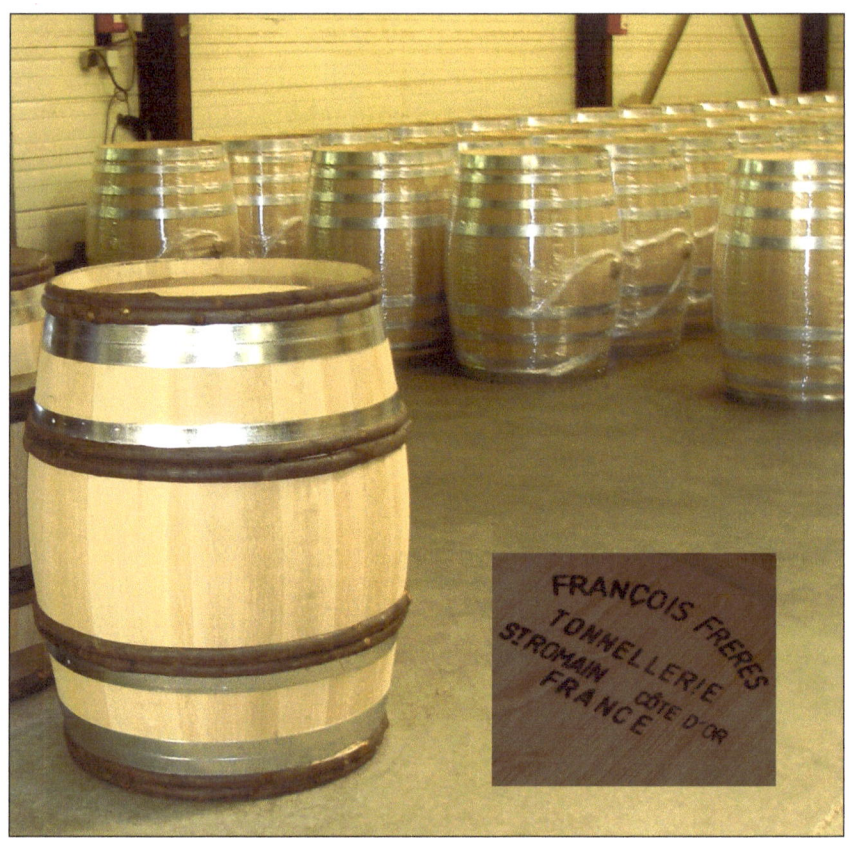

Tonnellerie François Frères – custom wine barrel makers

like northern California to me. The air was hot and smelled like grapes. Crickets serenaded us as we rolled alongside Le Rhoin, a nearby stream with picturesque, creekside campgrounds and suburban estates. Old stone buildings were numerous. In the heat, we were soon enveloped in swarms of gnats flying everywhere and attracted to the sweat beaded on our arms and legs. Our first ride in La Bourgogne had turned into a scenic 'bug fest'!

That evening we met Max Gigadet from François Frères in Beaune at *Ma Cuisine* for another fine French meal. Of course, many dinners might seem superb in the moment but this entire experience was exceptional. Max had made reservations and we were greeted by the proprietors, husband and wife Pierre and Fabienne Escoffier,[64] who also doubled as sommelier and chef. Both were wonderful hosts and friendly nice people. Gazpacho, bread and olives were served while we looked over the country style menu and a wine list with a mind blowing *20,000* choices! Naturally, we spent the next two hours enjoying the pleasant ambiance and delicious regional cuisine of the Bourgogne.

---

64. M. and Mme. Escoffier continue to successfully operate *Ma Cuisine* in Beaune.

The dining itself was like consuming art – the food was as beautiful to look at as it was delicious to eat. There was absolutely no rush to finish our meal. The aromas and flavors of my beef medallions with potatoes, string beans and mushrooms in a red wine sauce were delightful and satisfying. Max selected our dinner wines from 2003, considered an excellent year in this appellation of over 2000 domaines. I was being treated to an exquisite meal and the memorable opportunity of drinking premier wines from some of the most highly regarded producers in the Bourgogne region. Max paired a *Clos de la Justice,* pinot noir with our dessert – a ripened *fromage èpoisses*, fresh fruit and mint.

After returning to our hotel I checked the tour news. Australian Robbie McEwen had won the sprint at the Tour's lumpy 229 km Stage 2 in five hours, 36 minutes. Despite his injured arm, Thor Hushovd finished third and reclaimed the *maillot jeaune.*

Tuesday morning Frank went to meet Laurent Dufouleur of *Maison Tramier* and I explored Savigny-lès-Beaune – walking to some nearby higher ground where I could take in the view of surrounding environs. Three and four hundred year old stone buildings were everywhere and in use as residences or for other activities. The château and numerous churches were impressive and well maintained with full gardens, cemeteries and statuary. In the village, shops offering wine tasting and sales were located nearly every 50 meters (164 feet).[65]

Towards late afternoon we decided to take a bike ride along the *Route des Grands Crus* and somehow managed to avoid the swarms of gnats this time. Our route was a rolling, gradual 150 meter climb straight through a 'sea of green,' a limestone landscape of vineyards between Beaune and Villers-la-Faye. There was no breeze – the aroma of vineyards saturated the air. Traffic was light and not many people were out in the heat. We descended the escarpment from Villers–la-Faye through Chaux along a perfectly paved road with fast sweeping turns into the *Centre de Ville* in Nuits-St. George.[66] After an espresso and a quick look around we returned to Savigny along the main highway. It was straight and smooth, flat and fast, with a wide bike lane. *Le parcours était excellent!*

---

65. One meter equals 3.28 feet.
66. Nuits-St. George is the small, central village of the Côte d'Nuits in Burgundy.

Back at the hotel I was able to determine that German Matthias Kessler had ridden to a solo win in the Tour's hilly 216 km Stage 3, finishing in 4 hours, 58 minutes. Current World Champion, Belgian Tom Boonen had finished 4th, taking the *maillot jeaune.* Even with my tourist level understanding of French, I could see that the doping scandal was continuing to unfold as team managers and riders were questioned and some suspended or fired. The press was devouring 38 pages of evidence released two days earlier on July 2nd. Spanish racer Francisco Mancebo had abruptly announced his retirement.

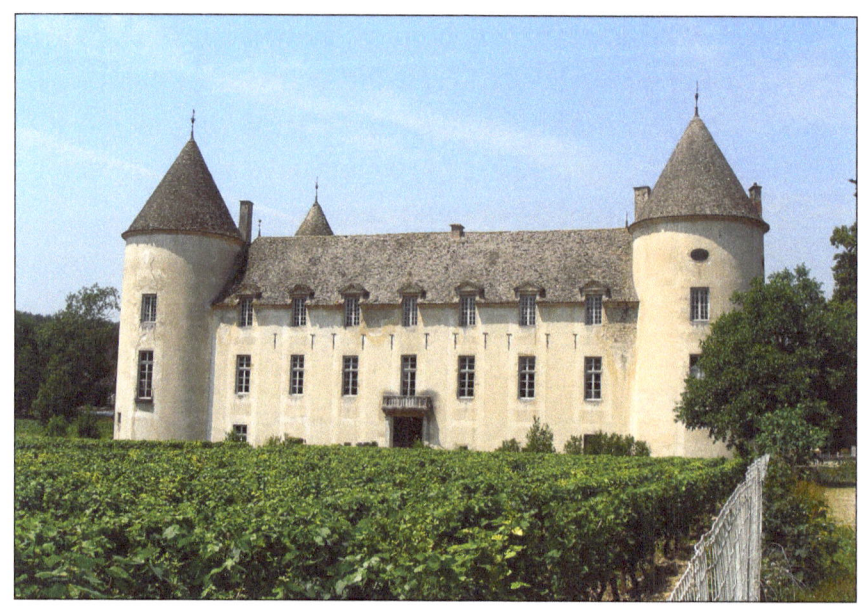

Château, Savigny-lès-Beaune

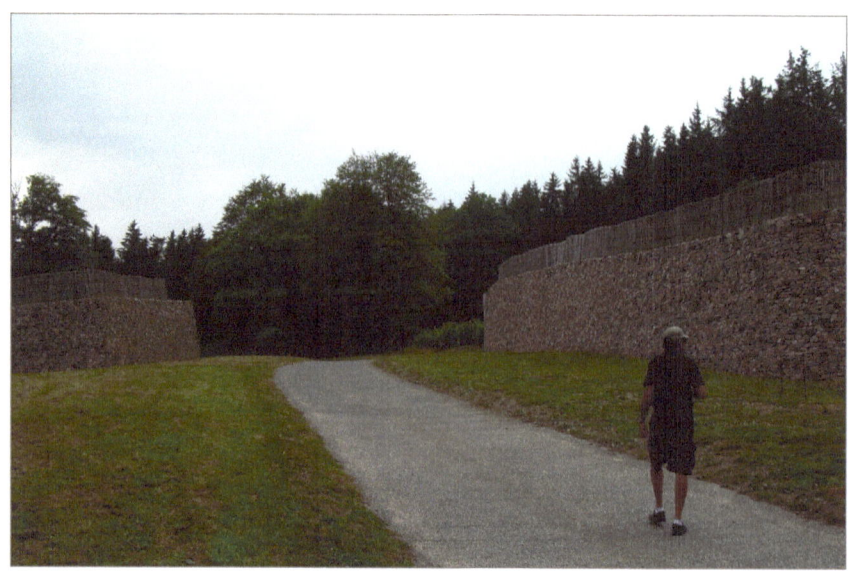

Reconstructed Iron Age ramparts at Bibracte

Rhône-Alpes

Wednesday, July 5th we traveled on from Beaune to the Rhône-Alpes where we'd made arrangements to stay in the tiny picturesque alpine village of Besse-en-Oisans, near Bourg d'Oisans and L'Alpe d'Huez.[67] Frank and I had planned another 'side trip' en route so we first drove west from Beaune to Bibracte[68] and hiked through an active archaeological site and reconstructed elements of a pre-Roman, Celtic settlement and ramparts, located near the summit of Mont Beuvray. The French government and international research community have long recognized the significance of this late Iron age site. Both support ongoing excavations and the Museum of Celtic Civilization, also located there. Bibracte was a fascinating place – well worth the drive – however, our enjoyable diversion put us directly on schedule to encounter some strong afternoon thunderstorms as we headed south through Grenoble towards the Alps.

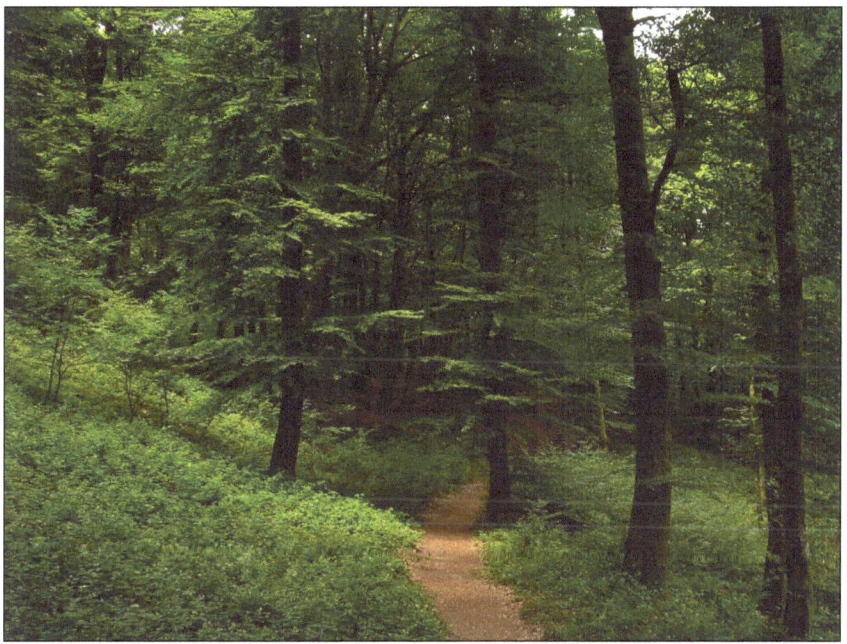

Wooded trail at the late Iron age Celtic settlement of Bibracte

---

67. L'Alpe d'Huez (elev. 1860 m/6100 ft) is the finishing point of perhaps the most legendary of all the high alpine climbs regularly included in the Tour de France. Bourg d'Oisans is the village near the base of the climb.

68. Bibracte is an extremely important 135 hectare (334 ac.) late Iron age site, a Celtic fortified hilltop settlement occupied by Romans in the first century BCE. Victorious in the Battle of Bibracte in 58 BCE, Julius Caesar later wrote his memoirs of the Gallic Wars while staying there. Under Gallo-Roman rule, the Celtic city of more than 30,000 inhabitants was rapidly abandoned and remained undisturbed until archaeological excavations were initiated during the late 19th century. Designated a Site of National Interest in 1989, a Roman basilica from 50 BCE found there is considered the oldest Roman monumental stone architecture in *non*-Mediterranean Europe. The Museum of Celtic Civilization and research center at Bibracte opened in the mid-1990s.

The blue sky above our beckoning backdrop of rugged Alpine terrain became ominous and black and we were soon enveloped in a severe downpour. The conditions made for several hours of slow going on the autoroute[69] but eventually the heavy rain abated and we arrived at Besse-en-Oisans around 7:30pm. There we met our beautiful, petite and pregnant host and her husband at the *Hôtel Alpin*. Crystal immediately served us an exquisite dinner consisting of Jerome's *filet mignon du porc* in a red wine mushroom sauce, with locally grown green beans and carrots, bread made in the village and local cheeses for dessert. I became even more convinced that the French prepare only food that is beautiful, fresh *and* delicious! We drank a bottle of Frank's newly acquired Burgundy red, vintage 1999 from *Maison Tramier.*

After dinner we watched France defeat Portugal in the semifinal World Cup match and met a crew of cyclists from Belgium, all there to ride in a major sportive event called *Le Marmotte*[70] the next Saturday. We chatted about the *Tour* and the unfolding doping scandal before saying *bonne nuit.*[71]

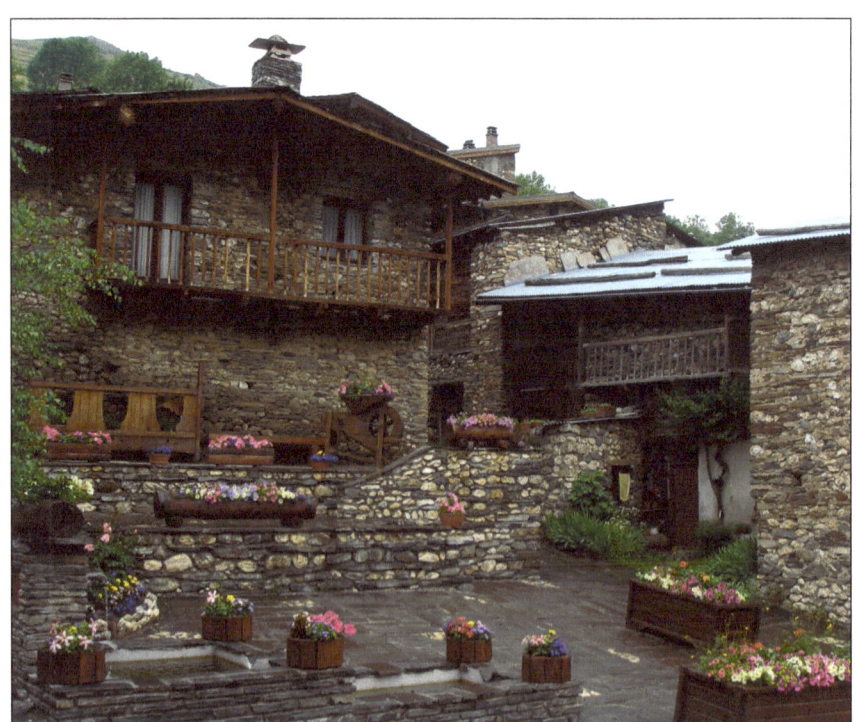

Hôtel Alpin, Besse-en-Oisans

---

69. The French equivalent of an 'interstate' highway in the United States.
70. Le Marmotte is considered the most difficult 'Sportive' ride in Europe – 6000 participants ride 175 km with 5000 meters of climbing, including the Col du Glandon (1924 m/6312 ft), Col du Galibier (2645 m/8677 ft), Col du Télégraphe (1566 m/5138 ft) and L'Alpe d'Huez, all in *one* day!.
71. Good night.

The Belgians spoke both English and French so they understood the emerging details of *Operación Puerto* more clearly than we did. But one thing was obvious to all of us – the scandal was exposing an undeniable systemic problem – a culture of doping in the professional peloton. After the long day we settled in at our *gîte*[72] and saw that Robbie McEwen had won another sprint in the Tour's flat 207 km Stage 4 in five hours. Tom Boonen had finished 4th and would remain in the *maillot jeaune.*

Geographically, Besse-en-Oisans was another truly amazing place. The 500 year old village had 1000 residents in the early 1900's – in 2006, there were just *eighty!* Perched on the southern side of the Massif Grandes Rouses, only stone buildings lined the narrow principal road that 'switchbacked' up the hill to this hamlet. No doubt the steep terrain and elevation make it a skier's paradise in winter. A cool thin layer of fog hung in the deep, narrow valley each morning. Muffled sounds of bells occasionally wafted uphill from where several cows grazed in the meadows below. Songbirds were numerous. Across the Riviére Romanche, the jagged, near 4,000 meter peaks and extensively folded sedimentary escarpments of the Massif des Écrins looked sublime.[73]

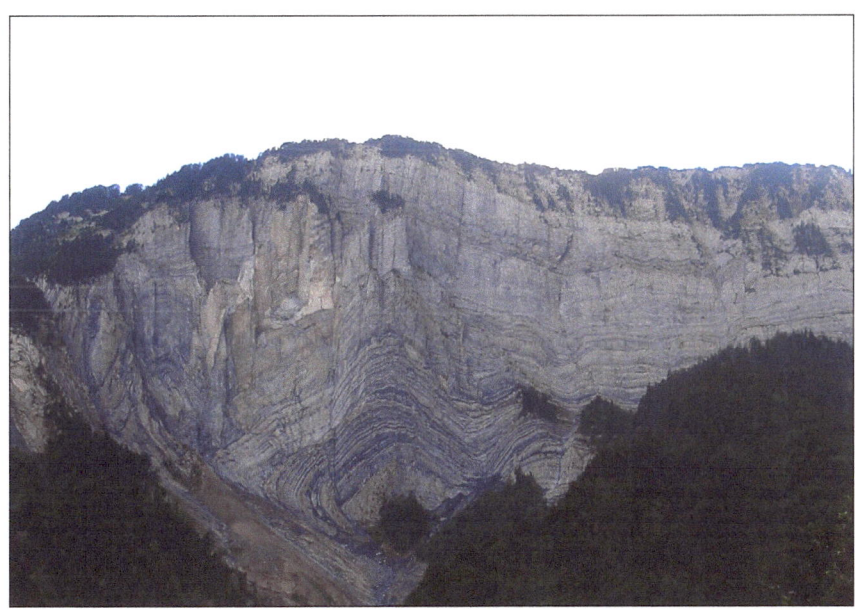

Sedimentary escarpment of the Massif des Écrins, Bourg d'Oisans

---

72. A *gîte* might be compared to a somewhat modest, rustic type of furnished vacation cottage.
73. Barre de Écrins (4,102 m /13,458 ft) and La Meijé (3,984 m /13,071 ft) are the two highest peaks in the Massif des Écrins.

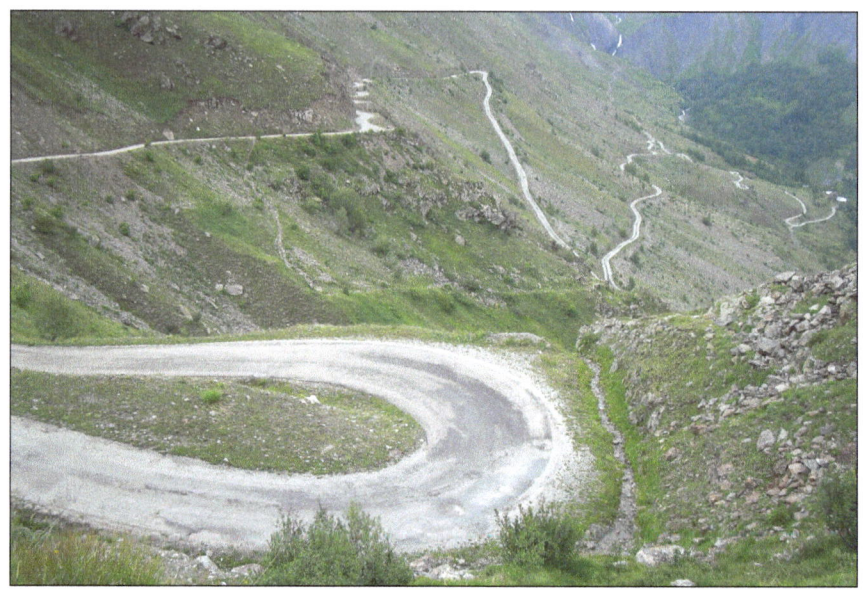

Switchbacks and rough pavement on the Rue de la Col de Sarenne

The next morning it was raining again. *C'est la vie*... we were destined to get wet on our 13 km climb to the Col de Sarenne,[74] a steady 7.5% ascent from another nearby hamlet, Clavans-en-Haute-Oisans. The rain showers increased near the summit. The narrow old road was rough with lots of loose gravel and sections where large stones had been installed in an uneven 'V-shaped' arrangement to provide drainage across the road. Frank and I rode steadily to the top, took our obligatory photos of the road monument and headed back down the mountain. The rain intensified, making the descent to Clavans slow and technical as we negotiated the uneven surface and numerous hairpin turns having no guard rails and a thirty meter cliff in places.[75] All things considered it was a good 90 minute 'rain' ride, steep and wet but not too cold or windy – no stiff hands or mishaps.

Back at the *gîte* we dried off, cleaned up the bikes and watched the Tour's Stage 5 action. The French television channel ITV broadcast live coverage of the Tour each day but unfortunately, didn't seem to display much race status information. The live commentators preferred to talk non stop instead! Of course, the word *'dopage'* was featured repeatedly. As the constant banter continued we were able to figure out that

---

74. The Col de Sarenne (elevation approx. 1,999 m/ 6,557 ft) is the 'back side'.
75. Approximately 90 feet. Racrs protested the inclusion of the Rue de la Col de Sarenne in the 2013 Tour de France.

Spaniard Óscar Freire had won the Tour's flat 225 km Stage 5 in five hours, 18 minutes. Tom Boonen was 2nd and would remain in the *maillot jeaune* for a third day.

Eventually the rain let up and we drove to Bourg d'Oisans, a bicyclist's 'Center of the Universe' all year long and *especially* in July! People were there from all over the world to ride in *Le Marmotte* or to see the Tour, which included the Stage 15 finish at the nearby L'Alpe d'Huez. We explored the *Centre de Ville* where streets are completely closed to auto traffic for the *entire month* of July. Nearly everyone in the heart of town was wearing cycling clothes – bicycles were everywhere. Four full service bike shops operated within a stone's throw of each other! Eager to practice his English, a mechanic at one of the shops told us they were doing brisk business with *Le Marmotte* riders who had suddenly decided they needed lower climbing gears installed before the weekend's event. The fresh alpine weather was cooler than in Paris or the Bourgogne but even in the shade of the late afternoon it felt comfortable – no jacket required.

After a late lunch it was time to do some 'recon' and drive the route to L'Alpe d'Huez. The idea of bicycling up this climb didn't appeal to me at *all!*[76] It was late afternoon as we drove passed hundreds of cyclists still steadily making their way up and down its 21 switchback turns.[77] At the top, the view towards the towering peaks of the Massif des Écrins was even more astonishing than it was from our *gîte* – 400 meters below in Besse. The Alpes are a geographer's dream – steep, bare sedimentary rock structures, folded and eroded into unimaginable shapes and forms during the last 80 million years. Frank's hard work the following day would be rewarded with a grand view!

We decided to drive 10 kilometers east on the rough rural road to the Col de Sarenne and then followed the same route we had bicycled that morning, descending to Clavans and Besse. The Route de la Col de Sarenne provided perhaps our most dramatic views of the verdant alpine grazing lands found in the highlands of the Plateau de Enparis. Situated at elevations of nearly two thousand meters, the flatter slopes are mostly treeless and covered with grasses punctuated by outcrops of bedrock.

---

76. Frank planned to do the legendary climb the next day while I followed in the car before meeting him at the summit.
77. 2,500 people *a day* ride this storied climb during the month of July!

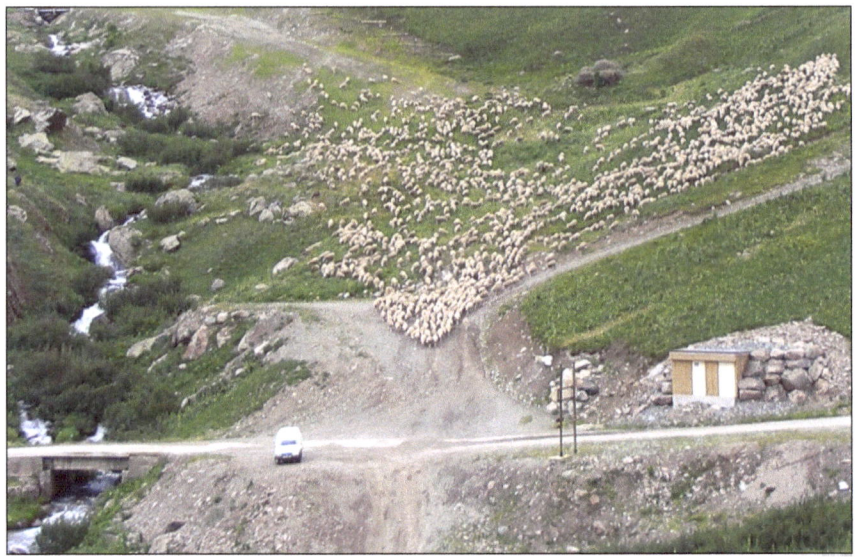

Sheep herd moving along the Rue de la Col de Sarenne

We stopped to take photos and through my camera's viewfinder I noticed a triangular patch of tan color off in the distance. Thinking that there was something on the lens, I took a cloth from my bag and suddenly realized that the speck had moved and gotten substantially larger. Far from being dust or light refraction, off in the distance I was seeing hundreds of sheep, packed tightly in a wedge shaped formation, following a single ram across the slopes below us. The texture of their long wool shimmered in the sunlight as they moved along in complete unison.

Friday we said goodbye to the unforgettable Besse-en-Oisans and drove down the mountain towards Bourg d'Oisans, where Frank took off on his bike and began his ascent of L'Alpe d'Huez. As planned, I followed in the car, slowly passing several *hundred* cyclists. There were also numerous delivery trucks inching their way along in *both* directions. It was obvious that pedaling was only a part of what makes climbing L'Alpe d'Huez such a huge challenge.

Preparations for the finish of *Le Marmotte* on the coming weekend were also underway, adding to the 'stop and go' driving conditions. The rain held off but the air was hot and heavy with the odors of exhaust and overheated brakes. I was glad to be Frank's support and not riding. When I reached the resort and parked it was quite a 'zoo' – the weekly local market and *Le Marmotte* cycling expo were happening. Both were crowded. Once Frank arrived and rested a bit we tracked down double espressos and quickly 'hit the road.'

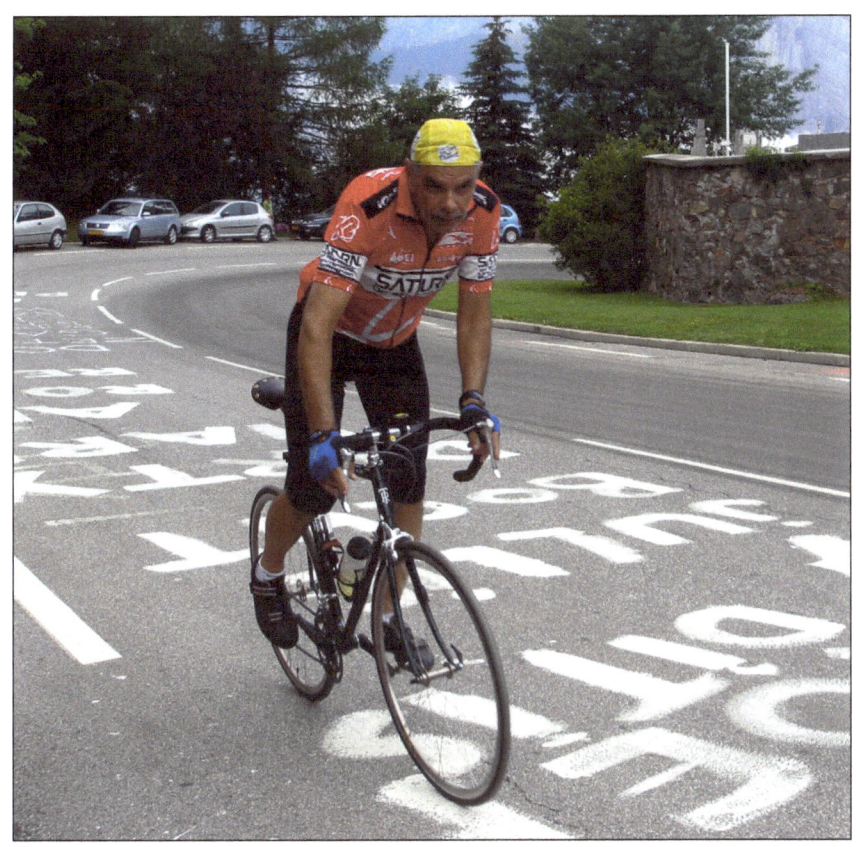

Frank Varvaro climbing the L'Alpe d'Huez

We headed down the mountain to Bourg d'Oisans, then over the Col du Glandon and Col de la Croix de Fer to our next destination – St. Jean de Maurienne in Savoie. Like Bourg d'Oisans, St. Jean de Maurienne is a haven for cycling and cyclists, especially during July. The Tour would pass through the town *twice* in 2006, on July 19th and 20th. Bicycles were everywhere. There were numerous local exhibits on *Tour de France* history, especially regarding the Col du Télégraphe and Col du Galibier, both nearby historic *HC* climbs of the Tour.[78] All over town we saw the news – Robbie McEwen had won his third sprint on the Tour's flat 189 km Stage 6 in four hours, 10 minutes. Tom Boonen finished 3rd and would keep the *maillot jeaune* for a fourth day.

Early Saturday morning we began our double dose of legendary climbs to the Col du Télégraphe and Col du Galibier by riding south on the departmental highway towards St. Michel de Maurienne. Immediately, we were overtaken by multiple groups of several *hundred* cyclists – all riding in *Le Marmotte*.

---

78. Depending on length and steepness, climbs are rated from 1 to 4, with *HC*, *Hors Catégorie*, (Beyond Categorization) being the 5th category, reserved for the very long and very steep climbs included in the Tour.

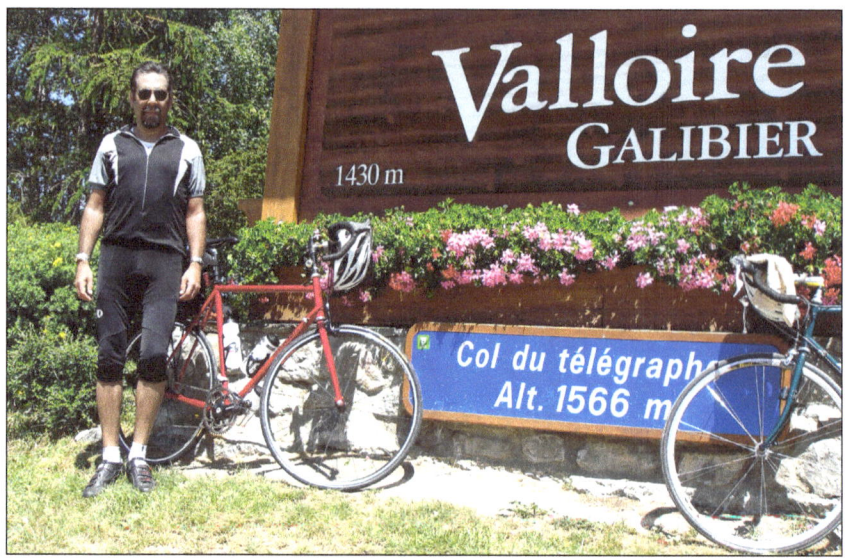

At the Col du Télégraphe

Frank caught the middle of the pace line in the second large group, while I was more comfortable drifting back in the *sea* of so many cyclists – some not so courteous.

It turned out that there were *three* large groups that caught up with us on the way to St. Michel de Maurienne. There the two of us began our 12 km (7.5%) ascent of the Col du Télégraphe. The groups strung out steadily but there were still many riders to contend with. Support cars, motorcycle escorts and medical vehicles also climbed slowly up the road. Volunteers at the support stops gave water to everyone – not just registered riders. It was already hot – most riders hung their helmets on their handlebars for the climb, as did we. The two of us reached the Col du Télégraphe about noon. After a brief rest and pictures Frank continued on to complete another 23 km, 9% climb to the summit of the Col du Galibier.

I stayed at the Col du Télégraphe, rested and watched the nonstop cycling action. I chatted with several Canadians and a couple from England as the main glut of riders rolled through. The afternoon had become unbearably hot and I witnessed a rider 'red line'[79] badly... he had reached the summit but pulled to the roadside immediately and began to sneeze uncontrollably. Soon he was lying on the ground and crews quickly came to his assistance. Eventually medics gave him saline intravenously to

---

79. Suffer symptoms of heatstroke.

stabilize him but he began to shiver and shake – panting. Within thirty minutes he and his bicycle were on their way down the mountain… in an ambulance. Heatstroke is no joke!

Frank returned in less than two hours. He rested while I told him about the 'red lined' rider and then the two of us then began our descent. Any remaining *Le Marmotte* riders were headed the opposite direction so there were far fewer bikes to contend with on our way down. Once we reached *St. Michel* de Maurienne, we stopped for water and then returned to *St. Jean* de Maurienne along the flat, departmental highway. The wind had picked up and we were 'treated' to our first persistent headwind. Frank was spent and tucked in behind me as I pushed into the wind for 13 km. It was 'mission accomplished' for both of us!

Back in St. Jean de Maurienne we cleaned up the bikes and watched coverage of Ukrainian Sergei Honchar, winning the Tour's flat 52 km Stage 7 time trial in just over an hour and taking the *maillot jeaune* from Tom Boonen. The USA's Floyd Landis finished one minute behind and took 2nd, also moving up into second place in the overall GC. A former teammate of Lance Armstrong[80] during his infamous run of seven *Tour de France* 'victories,' Landis was immediate target for suspicious fans and particularly the French sports press, who were steadily publishing stories about the *Operación Puerto* firings and interrogations going on. At the time, I felt like it was just *my* reaction but something about Landis seemed odd. Wearing his team cap backwards during interviews only accentuated his quirky expressions and demeanor.

Around six pm we stepped out to find a restaurant and settled on *Le Parenthese* where after a couple of beers I enjoyed a salmon salad and *tagliatelli a gambas*. Frank had filet mignon, roasted potatoes and vegetables. We had both earned a full meal. Dessert was also *très bien* – lemon, apricot and banana sorbet – combined. We smoked Cuban cigars after dinner and strolled back to the hotel, reflecting on how well the first ten days of the trip had gone and how it seemed that everywhere we went – the sorbet was something special!

---

80. Armstrong was eventually stripped of all seven of his Tour de France wins and received a lifetime ban from racing after Floyd Landis exposed the US Postal Service team's 'industrial-scale' doping program in 2010.

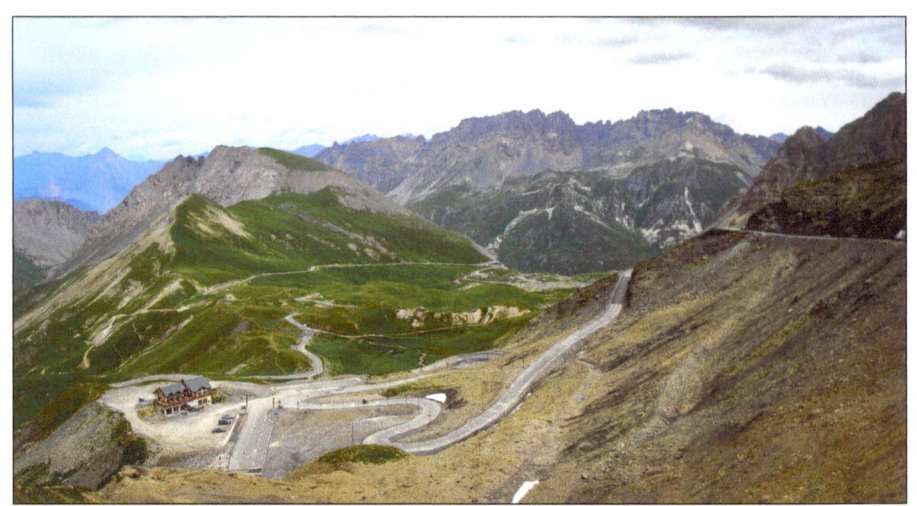
Rue du la Col de Galibier, Rhône Alpes

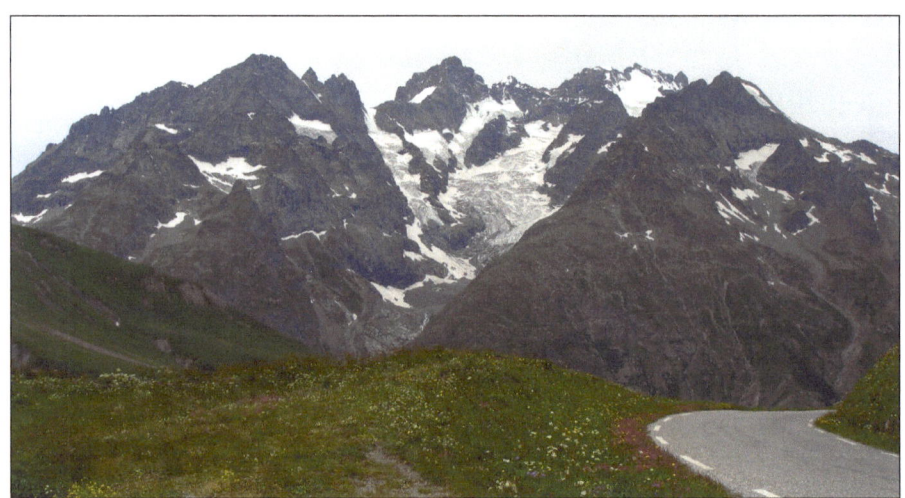
Les Pics du Combeynot and the Col du Lautaret, Hautes-Alpes

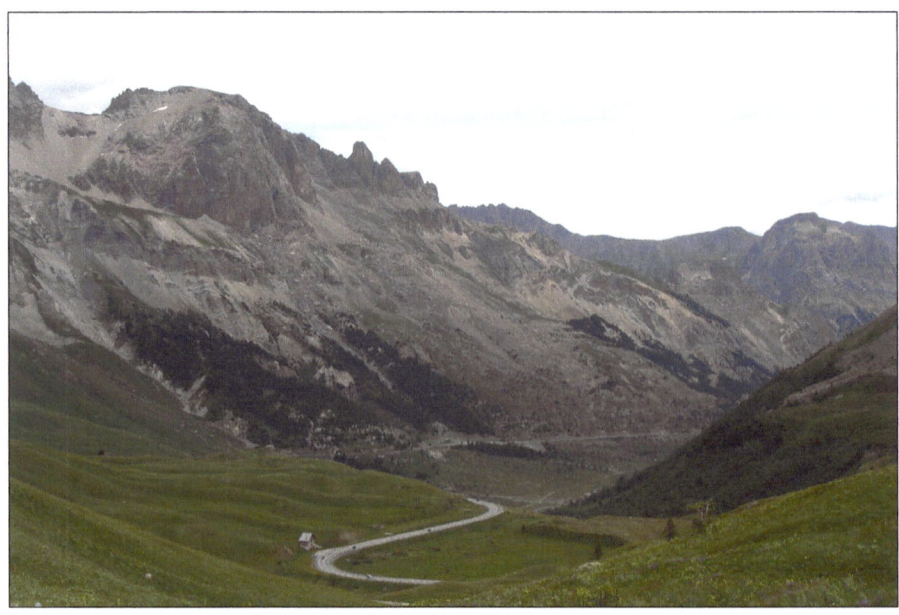
Departmental Road 1091 to Briançon, Hautes-Alpes

La Provençe

Sunday, July 9th was the Tour's first rest day and a travel day for us. We left St. Jean de Maurienne and followed the same route that we'd ridden the previous day, passing the Col du Télégraphe and continuing over the Col du Galibier. Frank had accomplished an *epic* feat to climb both the Galibier and Télégraphe together in the extreme heat... and doing so after climbing L'Alpe d'Huez and the Col de Sarenne the previous two days! We stopped for photos at the road elevation monument and then descended over the Col du Lautaret [81] to Briançon – a popular alpine resort to the south. People seemed to be on holiday – cyclists, motorcycles, cars and campers streamed steadily into the mountains.

We headed towards Gap and our next destination – La Provençe – first descending south from Briançon along the Riviére Durance towards Mont Dauphin. There were still majestic high mountains all along this glaciated valley – enough expansive vistas of hundred million year old sedimentary rocks to impress any geologist. At Mont Dauphin, the confluence of the Riviére Durance and the Riviére Guil sits below an imposing late 17th century château and fortified village built on a high promontory there.[82] The perimeter stone wall of this UNESCO site is completely intact and visible from a long distance.

We continued southwest through Savines-le-Lac where large dams have been built, creating the expansive blue-green Lac de Serre-Ponçon. Boaters, wind surfers and parasailors were numerous on the water. We crossed the lake at Pont de Savines and continued through Gap. Though still surrounded by thousand meter peaks the region felt different, more arid and southerly. By afternoon we were in Haute-Provençe.[83]

La Provençe is an amazing place for many reasons. The interesting and impactful human history and culture of this area is undeniable but it was immediately evident that the natural environment and geology of the region create an attractive, welcoming backdrop for life in the region. The landscape's natural palette is inspiring – it's easy to see why Cezanne, Van Gogh and many other artists have chosen to live and paint in Provençe.

---

81. Elevation 2000 m (6562 ft)
82. The fortified town was built 1000 meters above the Riviére Guil from 1693-1700 by Sébastien Vauban, chief military engineer for King Louis XIV. Mont Dauphin was listed as a UNESCO World Heritage Site in 2008
83. The northern part of Provençe.

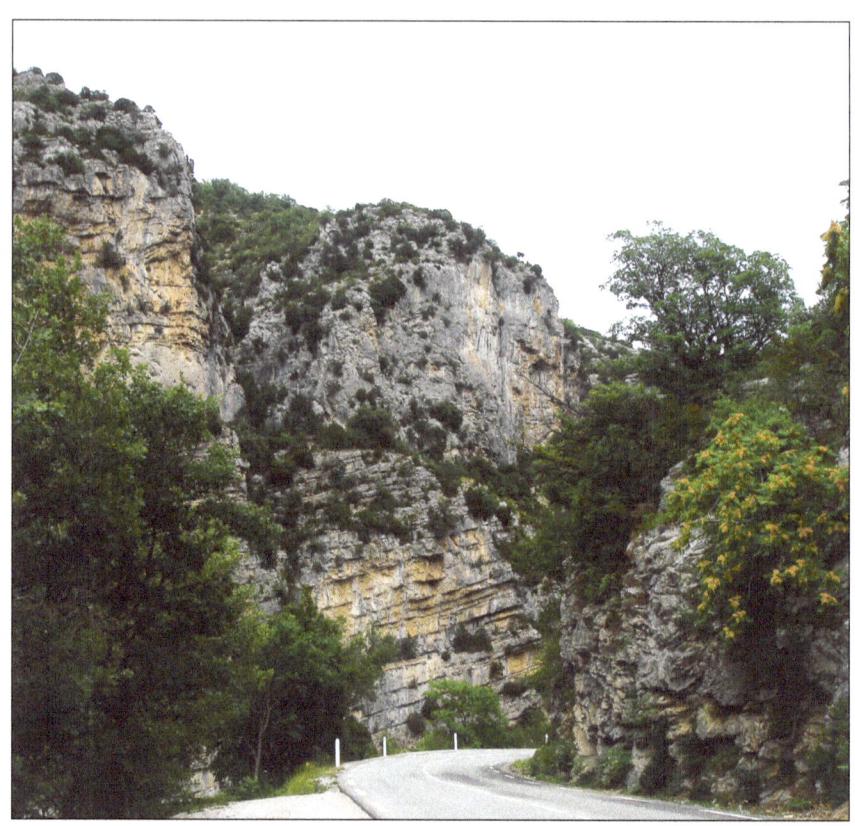

Following the gorge of the Riviére Aigues, Haute-Provençe

Long before Romans made it their *Provincia* the entire region was part of a Mesozoic-era sea.[84] The bedrock is made up of sedimentary layers like the Alps and Pyrenees, however, the area we now call Provençe was faulted and folded differently when the Earth's crustal plates shifted and collided – 100 million years ago – creating the adjacent high mountains. There are rugged mountains in Provençe but the terrain is dominated by extensive plateaus and moderate slopes carved into the limestone and clay river valleys. Natural oxides of iron have colored the topsoil red, yellow and orange.

We crossed into the next Department at Verclause following the Riviére Aigues through its narrow gorge. The air temperature reached 90°F (32°C) by mid afternoon. Like sirens, cicadas along the riparian corridor sang loud and steadily throughout the *Parc Naturel Régional des Baronnies Provençales,* where numerous caves host vultures roosting in the near vertical cliff faces lining the river on both sides. Regardless of orientation, the rock strata

---

84. 252 million to 66 million years ago.

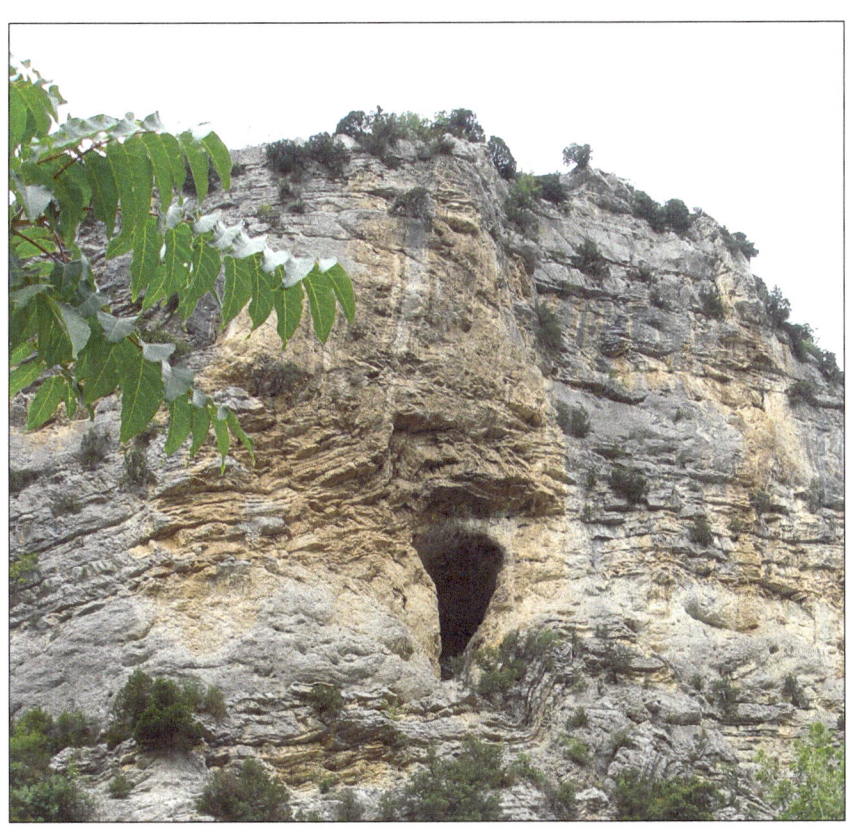

Limestone cave in the Parc Naturel Régional des Baronnies Provençales

revealed complex, convoluted folds like those we'd seen at the Massif des Écrins. The change in geography became even more obvious – The highest peaks were now in the two thousand meter range, the soils stony. Gentler slopes were dotted with olive, apricot and cherry trees. Of course, there were vineyards – with Grenache, Syrah, Mourvèdre and Carignan grapes as opposed to the Chardonnay and Pinot Noir grown in the north.

We turned south at Nyon. The landscape looked clearly Mediterranean with tile roofs everywhere and ochre-color buildings, older that those in Savoie and Oisans. The landscape was looked golden in the late afternoon sunlight. We arrived in Malaucène and immediately found lodgings in the center of town. The *Hôtel L'Origan* would be perfect for a weeklong stay. Besse-en-Oisans had been impressively old but Malaucène was much older.

The next day we explored the medieval part of Malaucène on foot. As in other parts of France, Celtic tribes lived here before the period of Roman domination. Two thousand year old Roman walls were later integrated into the *Cathédrale Saint-Michel,* built in the 14th century. The church's 400 year old organ is covered with gold leaf. [85] Just a short walk up a nearby hill there were Roman era cisterns built where a spring was tapped to bring water to the village. The spring was running strong and the cisterns were full.

Back at the hotel I determined that Frenchman Silvain Calzati had ridden alone 31 km to victory in the Tour's flat 181 km Stage 8, finishing in four hours, 13 minutes. Sergei Honchar finished with the chasing group and kept the *maillot jeaune.* Floyd Landis stayed in second place overall – one minute behind him.

Adding to the stream of daily racing and *Operación Puerto* news, Landis now revealed that he was planning to undergo hip surgery in the fall. Frank and I thought something about his announcement sounded strange but it was still easy to root for him in the moment. He was a second tier favorite doing well in a year when the first tier competition had been *disqualified* – an American racer who, like me, was facing hip surgery.[86]

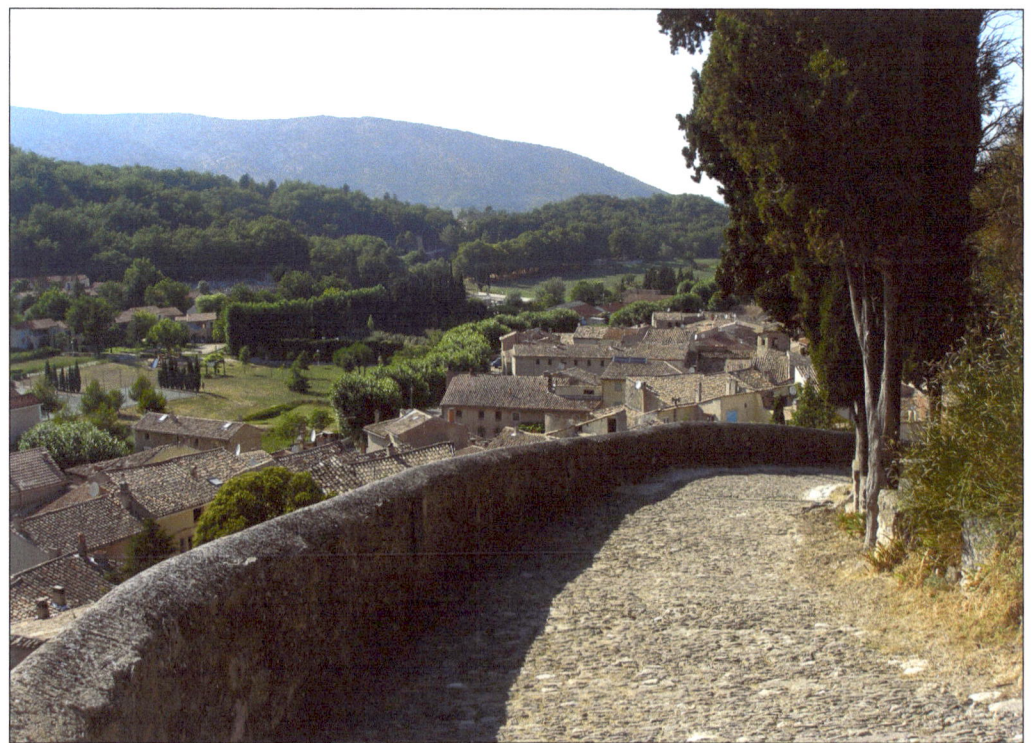

Cobbled street in the Cité Médievale, Malaucène, Provençe

---

85. Restored in the 1950's, it was made a national monument in 1970
86. After fracturing a hip in 1985, I was now expecting to need hip replacement surgery within a year or two.

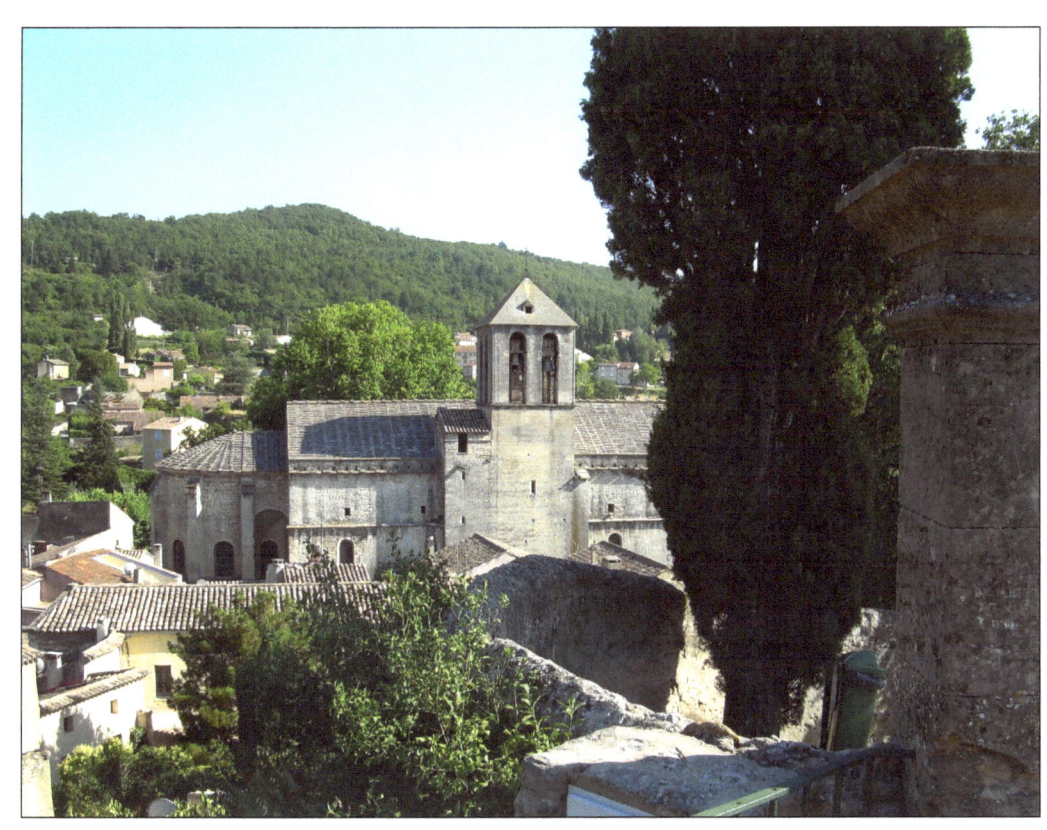

Cathédrale Saint-Michel, Malaucène, Provençe

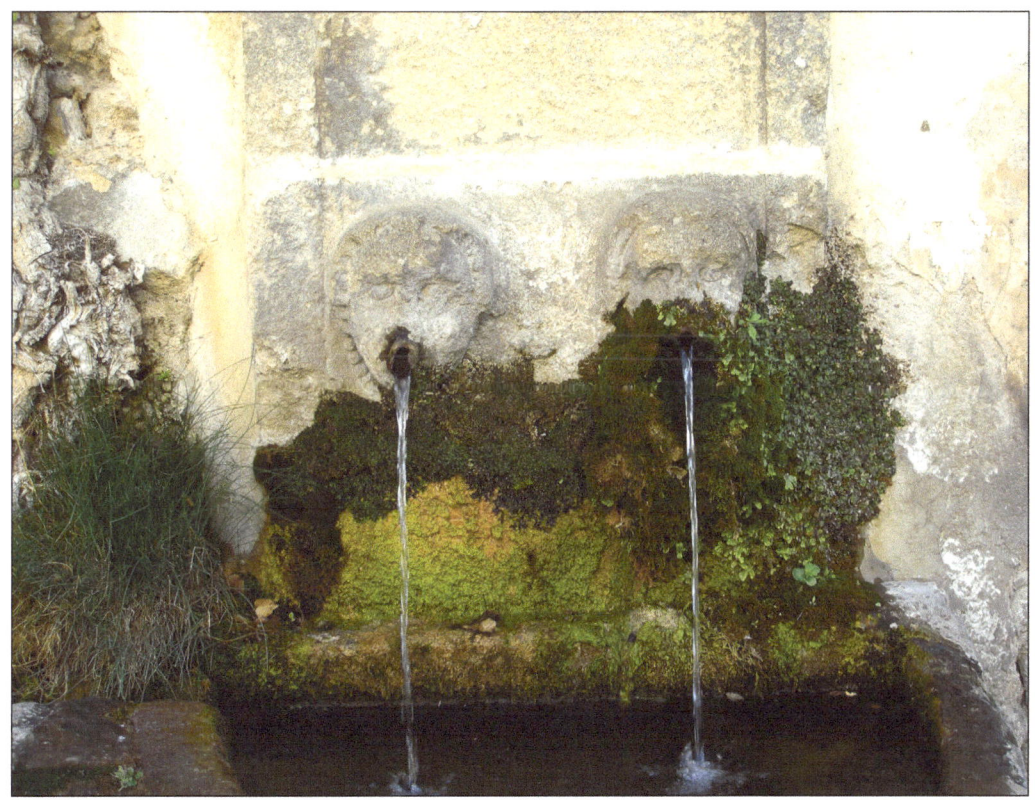

Spring-fed Roman fountain, Malaucène, Provençe

Tuesday was *'V-Day'* for us – the day we had chosen to ride to the top of the UNESCO Biosphere Reserve at Mont Ventoux,[87] a 21.5 km climb from Malaucène with many microclimates and exposed stretches of road.[88] A number of wooded sections provide some shade but we wisely began around 9 am before it got hot. The average gradient is 7.5% with some sections reaching 12%. It was tough on the ramps but otherwise very manageable with my 'compact crank' gearing.[89] All things considered – it was a straightforward climb and extraordinary cycling 'fun.' The 'slow going' made it easy to see some of Mont Ventoux's high diversity of plants, birds and animals.

The experience of riding such a historic climb of the *Tour de France* was steady motivation for the one and a half hour effort. I stopped just once for a short shade break at the Château Liotard near Mont Serein.[90] The last 5 km was a grind – with some wind, the full exposure of bare limestone above the tree line and an increasing gradient. But it went by quickly – I distracted myself with the Alpine poppies in bloom. Seeing the observation tower and knowing I was approaching the peak helped keep the legs turning. Despite hazy air below it was breezy and clear at the top.

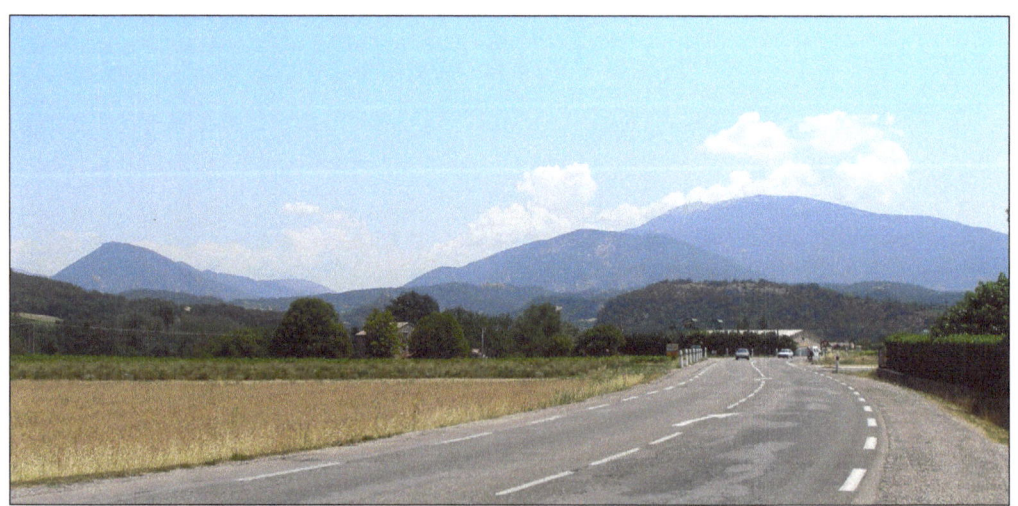

On the road from Malaucène to Mont Ventoux, the Giant of Provençe

---

87. Mont Ventoux (1,912m /6,273 ft), 'The Giant of Provençe, has been climbed in many editions of the Tour.
88. Malaucène's elevation is 365 m (1,198 ft), making the climb about 1,550 m (5,076 ft).
89. Chainrings:34/50; 10-speed freewheel with 13-26 tooth cogs.
90. Mont Serein is located about five kilometers from the peak of Mont Ventoux at an elevation of approx. 1,430 meters.

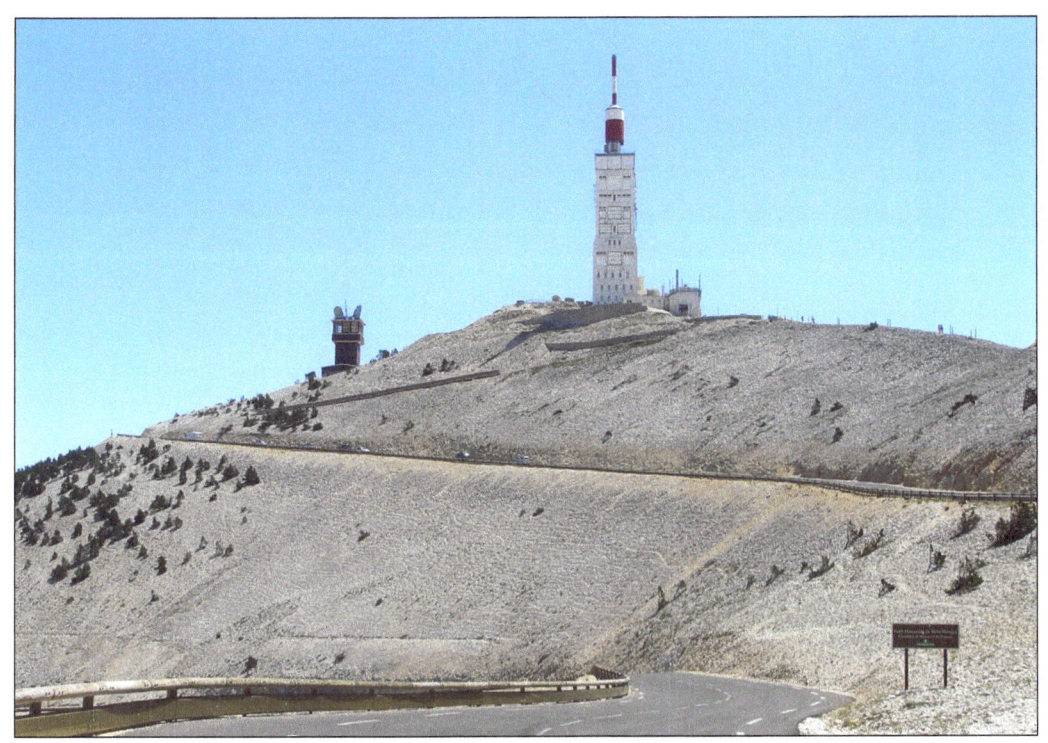

Approaching the summit of Mont Ventoux

The expansive panoramic views reminded me of Mount Diablo in northern California. I convinced myself that I was seeing the Alps, Pyrenees and Mediterranean Sea in my 360° view of the horizon.

As expected, the peak itself was crowded with cars, cyclists and hikers. Concessionaires sold fruit and candy in the parking lot at 'rip-off' prices. There was also a souvenir store where I bought three tiny bottles of Perrier – for *6 euros!* We took our obligatory photos near the Mont Ventoux monument and struck up a conversation with some people we heard speaking English. They turned out to be from Seattle, Washington and had friends there who were members of Frank's cycling club. It's a small *cycling* world, too!

We returned to Malaucène by reversing our route. It was a well deserved reward for all the climbing with a long fast descent following the uppermost section of hairpin turns. Back in Malaucène it felt nearly 100°F (38°C). It was still early so we cleaned up the bikes and watched the Tour's live broadcast. Spanish sprinter Óscar Freire won the flat 169 km Stage 9 in three hours, 35 minutes with Sergei Honchar remaining in the *maillot jeaune.* Floyd Landis was still in second place – a minute behind. That evening, the weather was perfect for dinner on the hotel restaurant's patio – we'd both earned our hearty

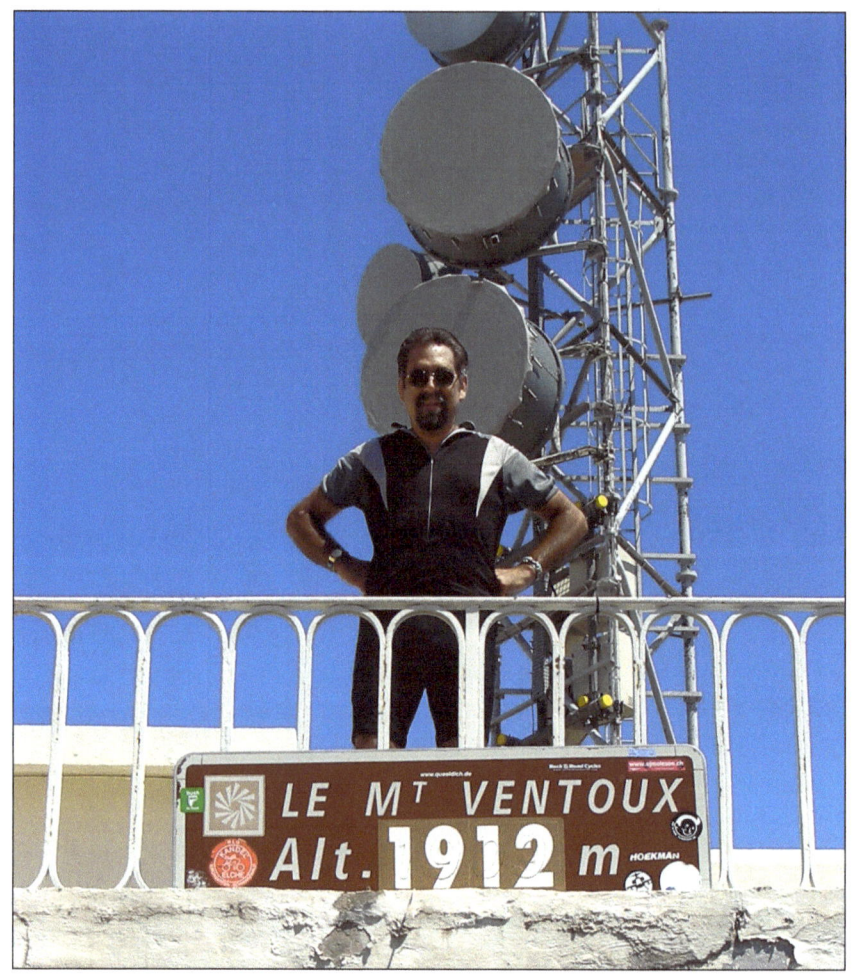

At the summit of Mont Ventoux

meal – sirloin steaks served Provençal style with truffle cream, roasted carrots and potatoes, a summer salad, Côte du Rhône red wine, with cheese and fresh fruit for dessert.

Wednesday was a logical rest day after our climb up the limestone 'giant' the previous morning. We took it easy and watched the Tour's live broadcast again. Our fellow countryman was in second place, and the race was now entering the Pyrenees Mountains, where numerous difficult climbs lay ahead. Spaniard Juan Mercado won the day's mountainous 191 km Stage 10 in four hours, 49 minutes. The peloton finished nearly *seven and a half minutes* behind Mercado and Frenchman Cyril Dessel took 2nd place, vaulting himself from 28th place into the *maillot jeaune!* Floyd Landis slipped to 5th place in the GC – four minutes, 45 seconds behind Dessel.

The next morning we rode the bikes south through the surrounding Rhône Valley wine country to the villages of Vacqueyras and Gigondas, then back to Malaucène via Vaisson-la-Romaine – a fifty kilometer clockwise loop around the regionally prominent and jagged peaks of the Dentelles de Montmirail.[91] Provençe is a seismically active area with rolling terrain and fault lines controlling the topography in parts of the region, which made for some 'lumpy' kilometers. We gradually climbed to Suzette and continued south, heading through Lafare and Beaume de Venise, then north to Vacqueyras and Gigondas on the western flanks of the Dentelles de Montmirail.

Both Vacqueyras and Gigondas are well known for their exceptionally fine Provençal wines. The combination of limestone soils, topography and proximity to the steep sided Dentelles de Montmirail creates a unique environment for the growing of noble red and white grape varieties. There is evidence of winemaking here two thousand years ago and it's clearly still going strong. We stopped at a local wine producer's cooperative in Gigondas and sampled some exquisite rosé while sitting below the 11th century Saint Catherine's church and castle ruins that overlook the small village.

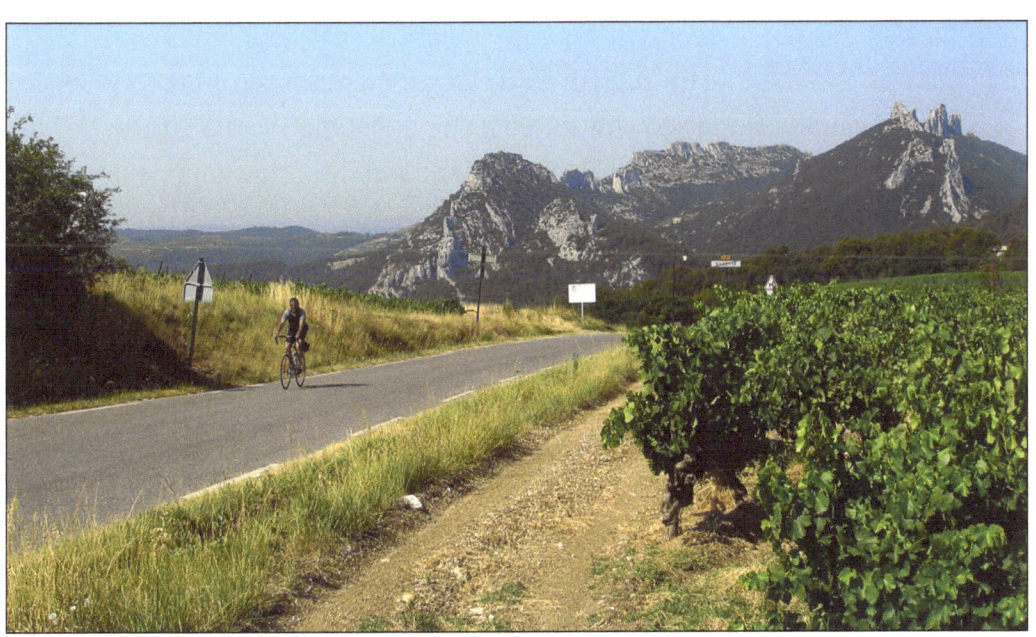

The Côte du Rhône: Dentelles de Montmirail, Provençe

---

91. A Jurassic period limestone formation, inclined vertically and eroded into a series of bare, craggy spires with peaks from 500 to over 700 meters. The area is popular with hikers, rock climbers and mountain bikers.

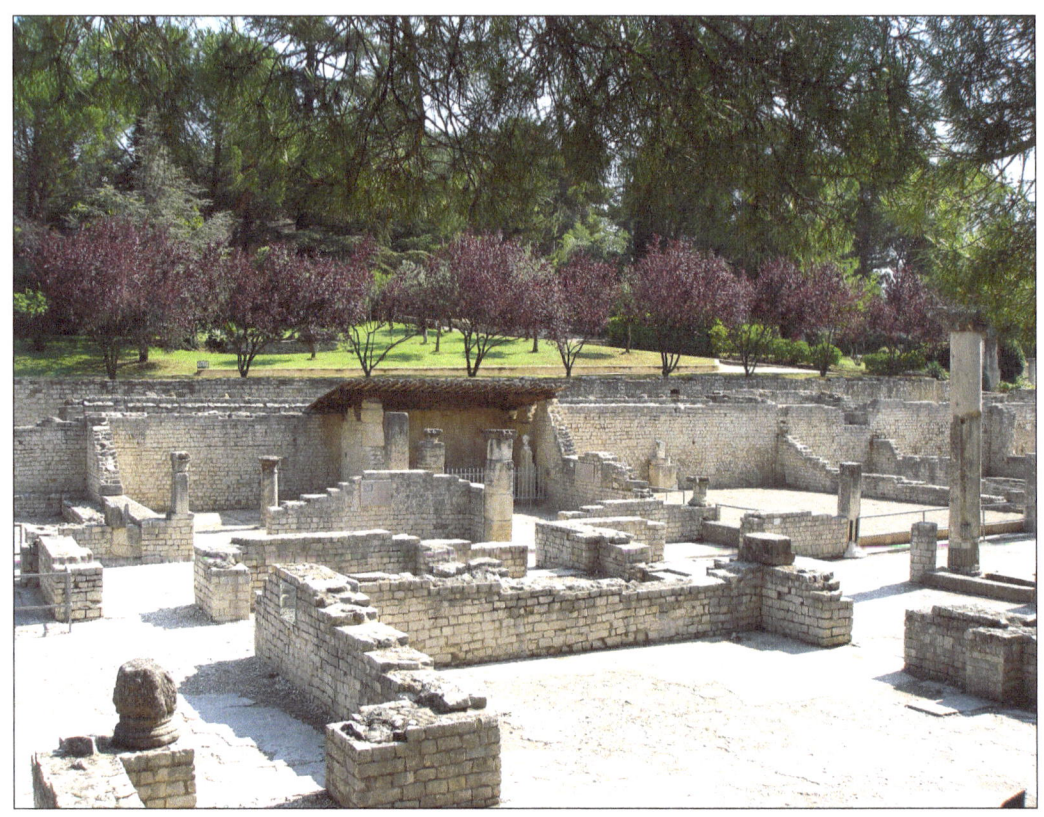

Remains of *Vasio Vocontiorum*, a 2nd century federated Roman city, Vaisson-la-Romaine, Provençe

We rode on to Vaisson-la-Romaine and climbed into the 14th century hilltop *Cité Médiévale.* Stone buildings built centuries ago were everywhere and remain in use as homes and shops. Descending through the old city gate we crossed a 1st century Roman bridge and continued a short distance to the largest archaeological site in France open to the public – the remains of *Vasio Vocontiorum,* a 2nd century federated Roman city.[92] There we were, silently walking our bikes through a vast Roman ghost town full of nobles' homes, artifacts and an amphitheater built two thousand years ago!

Afternoon showers commenced and we rode a wet but warm and flat ten kilometers further, as we returned to Malaucène. A bike cleaning session followed, along with a late lunch while watching the Russian Denis Menchov win the Tour's second mountainous 207 km Stage 11 in six hours, six minutes. Floyd Landis finished with him, four minutes, 45 seconds ahead of the peloton and took the *maillot jeaune* from Cyril Dessel! The yellow jersey had now changed wearers six times, en route to a new record of *ten!*

---

92. The well preserved Roman ruins at Vaisson-la-Romaine include a theatre, public bath foundations and the homes of nobles

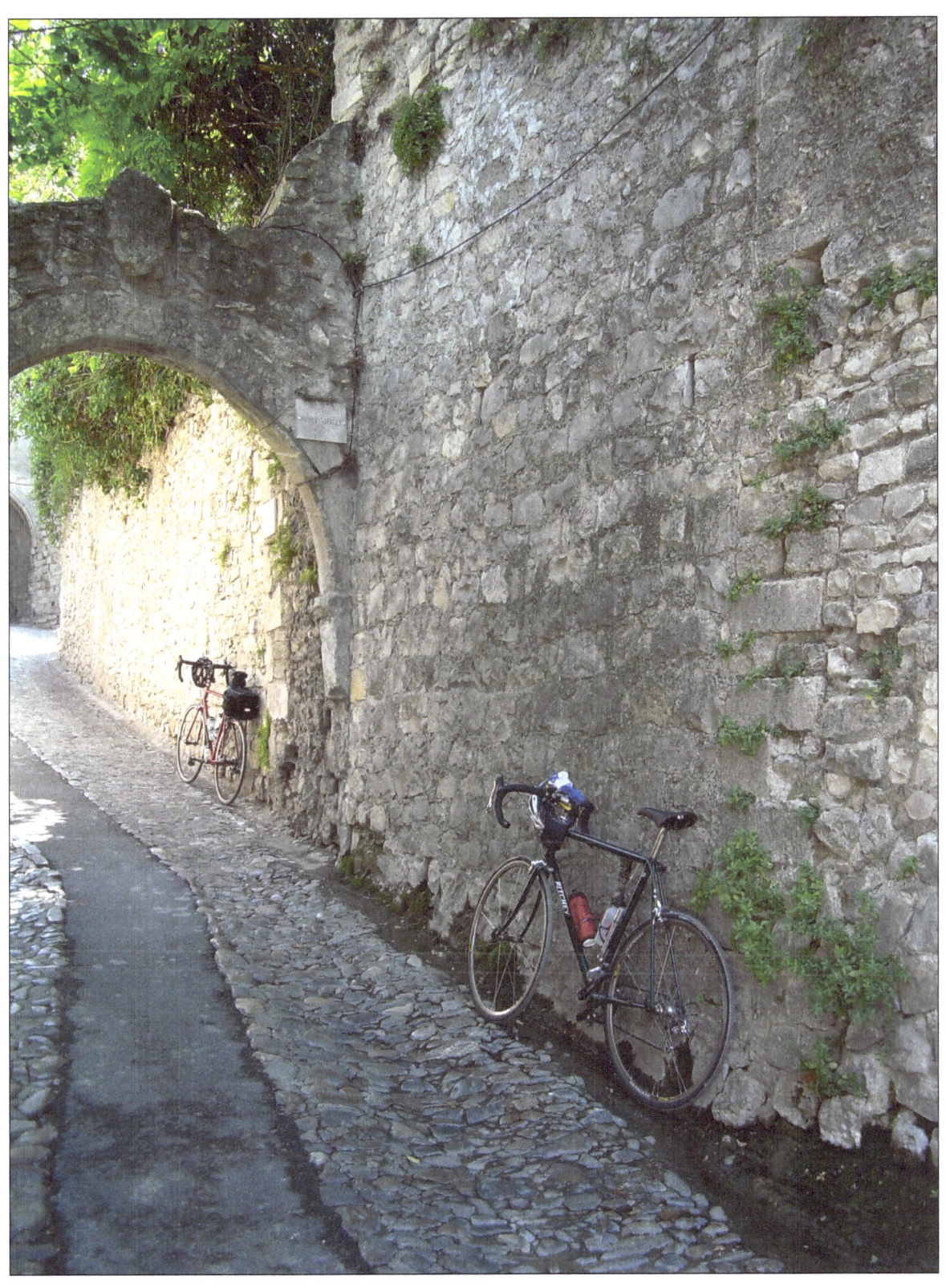

Portal to the 14th century Cité Médievale, Vaisson-la-Romaine, Provençe

In France, July 14th is called *Quatorze Juillet or Fête Nationale* – the National Holiday.[93] That Friday morning we set off to celebrate the day with a looping forty kilometer ride into the Vaucluse plateau wine country south of Malaucène. We staged the ride from Venasque,[94] one of the earliest medieval hilltop villages in France. The first fifteen kilometers took us into the *Forêt de Venasque* through a narrow limestone gorge with near vertical cliff walls, caves and a 4% grade – then over the Col de Murs[95] to our second hilltop village of the day – Murs. After a quick stop to look at its 15th century château, we descended further amidst vineyards and stunning blue fields of blooming lavender.

We continued downhill to Gordes – the day's third and, perhaps, most picturesque fortified hilltop village. Its church, 16th century castle and stone buildings were nestled together around a small plaza perched near the edge of the Vaucluse plateau. I imagined how Gallo-Roman medieval chieftains must have valued the commanding view of the countryside below during times of attempted invasions. We took our break in the plaza and met some touring Australian cyclists planning to ride Mont Ventoux and L'Alpe d'Huez. Our climb out of Gordes took us past the 12th century Abbaye Sénanque, an active Cistercian

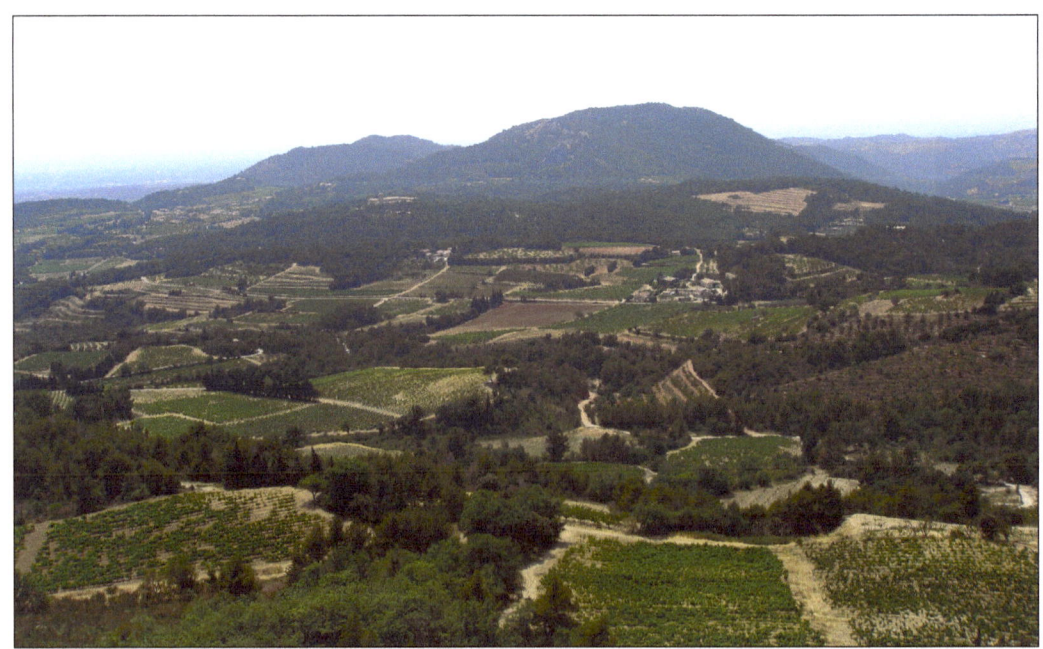

Vineyards in the Vaucluse Plateau, Provençe

---

93. *Bastille Day*, July 14, 1789 is only one of several important July dates in French history.
94. First built in the 6th century, Venasque is the site of an early medieval baptistery and an 11th century Romanesque church.
95. Elevation 628 m (2,060 ft).

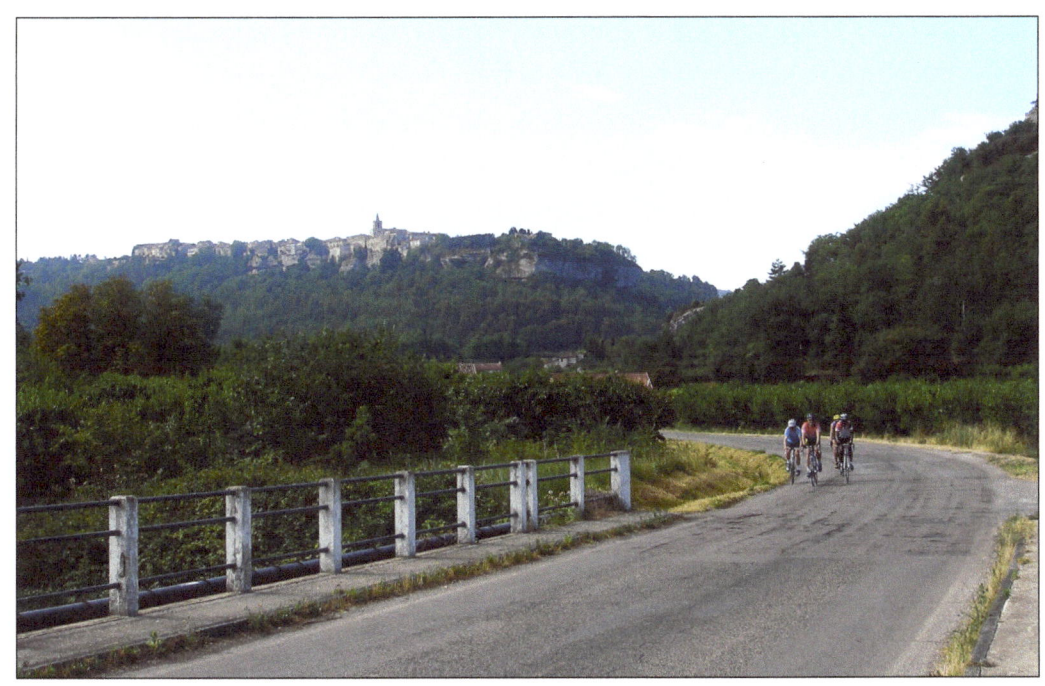

On the road near the medieval city of Venasque, Provençe

monastery where monks take vows of silence and cultivate seemingly endless fields of lavender. Butterflies were numerous all along the entire return to Venasque.

Clouds had gathered and showers began as we reached Venasque and drove back towards Malaucène. Rain continued into the warm evening – only letting up about 10 pm. Undeterred, the local holiday fireworks display began soon after and while modest, the show was something special. Everyone from the village seemed to be out enjoying it. The finale went on for quite a while – with a perfect backdrop of the clear, night sky.

After the fireworks, Frank turned in and I strolled around the *Centre de Ville*, returning to find *Ricky Novak* and his band rockin' and rollin' on the temporary stage set up *directly below my hotel room!* Dozens danced to his covers of American 1950s and 60s hits like *Rock Around The Clock, La Bamba* and so forth. Other pop hits like Sinatra's *I Did It My Way* were sung in French! Prince's *1999* and Marvin Gaye's *What's Goin' On?* sung in English with a heavy French accent sounded especially cheesy. Then there was *La Macarena!*

Nevertheless, it was memorable fun being in Provençe to witness the National Day festivities. The people watching was superb – the music... not so good. Eventually I retired to my room and watched a rebroadcast of the Tour's rolling 212 km

Stage 12, where Russian Yaroslav Popovytch rode the final 8 km solo to win in four hours, 35 minutes. Floyd Landis remained in the *maillot jeaune*, holding a thirty second lead over Cyril Dessel in the GC. The *Quatorze Juillet* revelry continued until 2:00 am!

Although one of the Tour Directors, Cristian Prudhomme, was now making public comments about doping amidst the constant drumbeats of *Operación Puerto*, it was still easy to focus mostly on the racing. It had been exciting so far and a USA racer was now in the overall lead!

Saturday morning Frank and I headed north to Montélimar to watch the finish of the 230 km Stage 13, longest of the 2006 Tour, *in person!* We checked out the village and then walked to the finish line where we watched the race action projected on a jumbo screen. The air temperature was 104°F (40°C) and the crowd – absolutely huge.

It was impossible to get close enough to photograph the race finish – I settled for images of the awards ceremony... Germany's Jens Voight won the day's rolling Stage 13 in five hours, 25 minutes. Spanish racer, Óscar Pereiro took second, vaulting himself from *46th* place into the *maillot jeaune!* It was a long hot day – over 150 racers finished nearly *thirty minutes* behind Voight. One of them – Floyd Landis – had lost the yellow jersey and now sat in second overall... one minute, 29 seconds behind Pereiro.

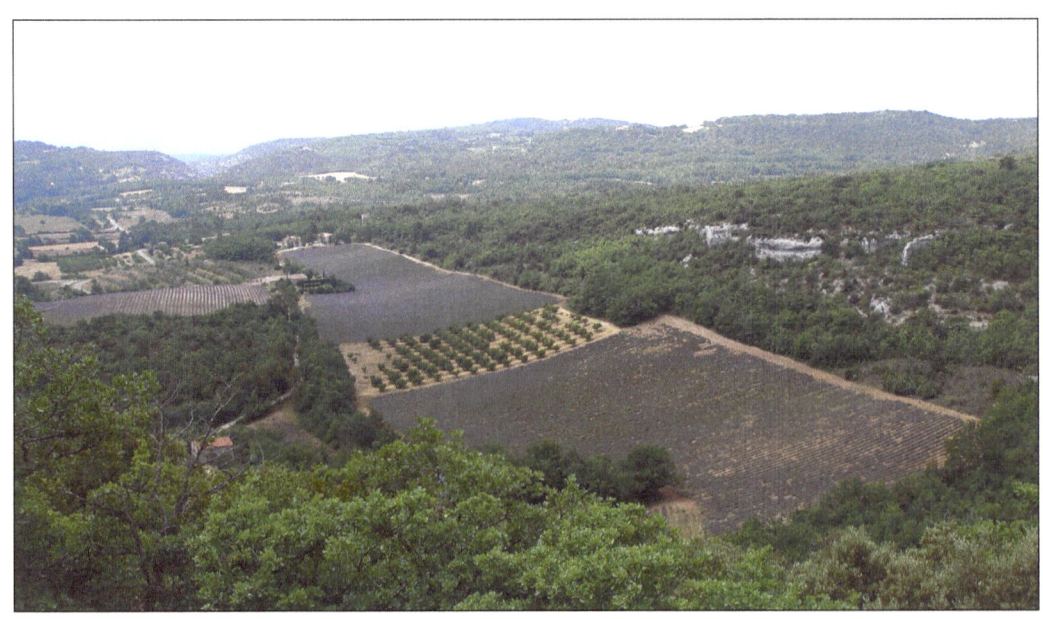

Lavender fields near the 12th century Abbaye Sénanque

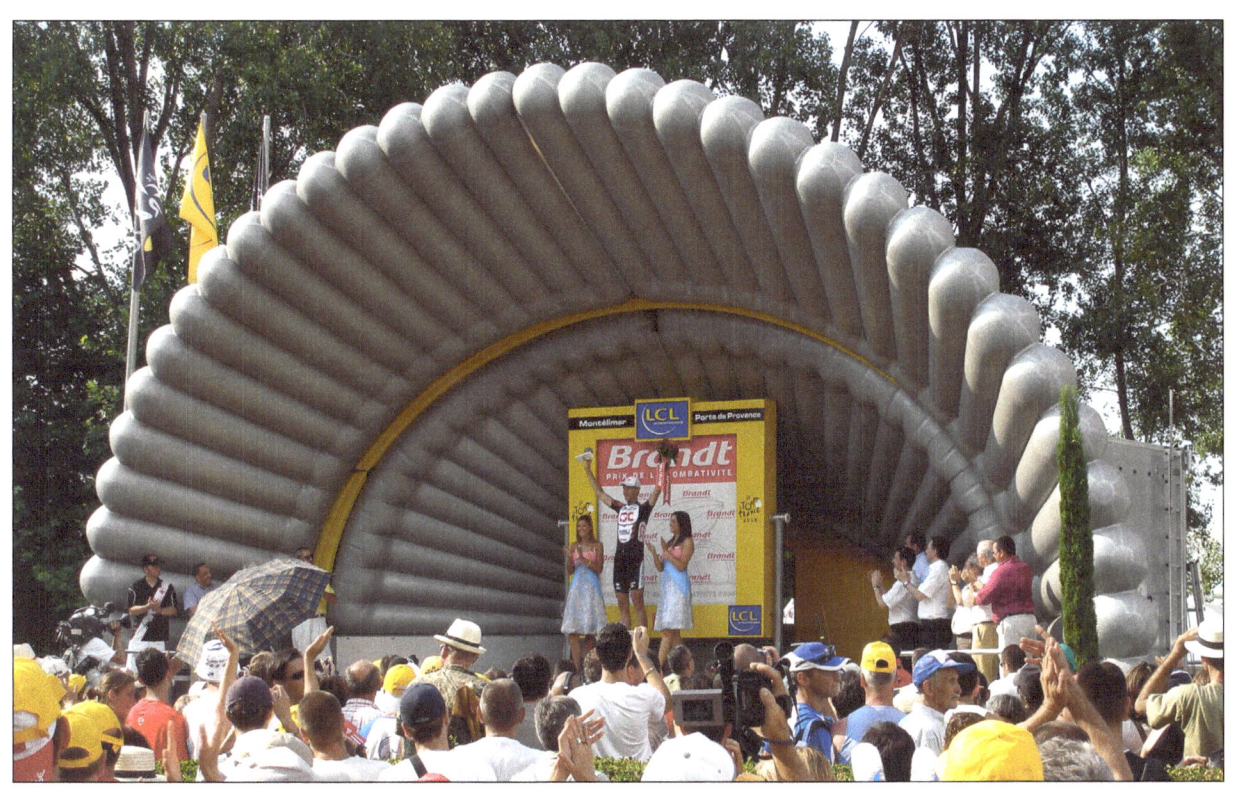

German Jens Voight, winner of the 230 Km (143 mi.) Stage 13 of the 2006 Tour de France, Montélimar

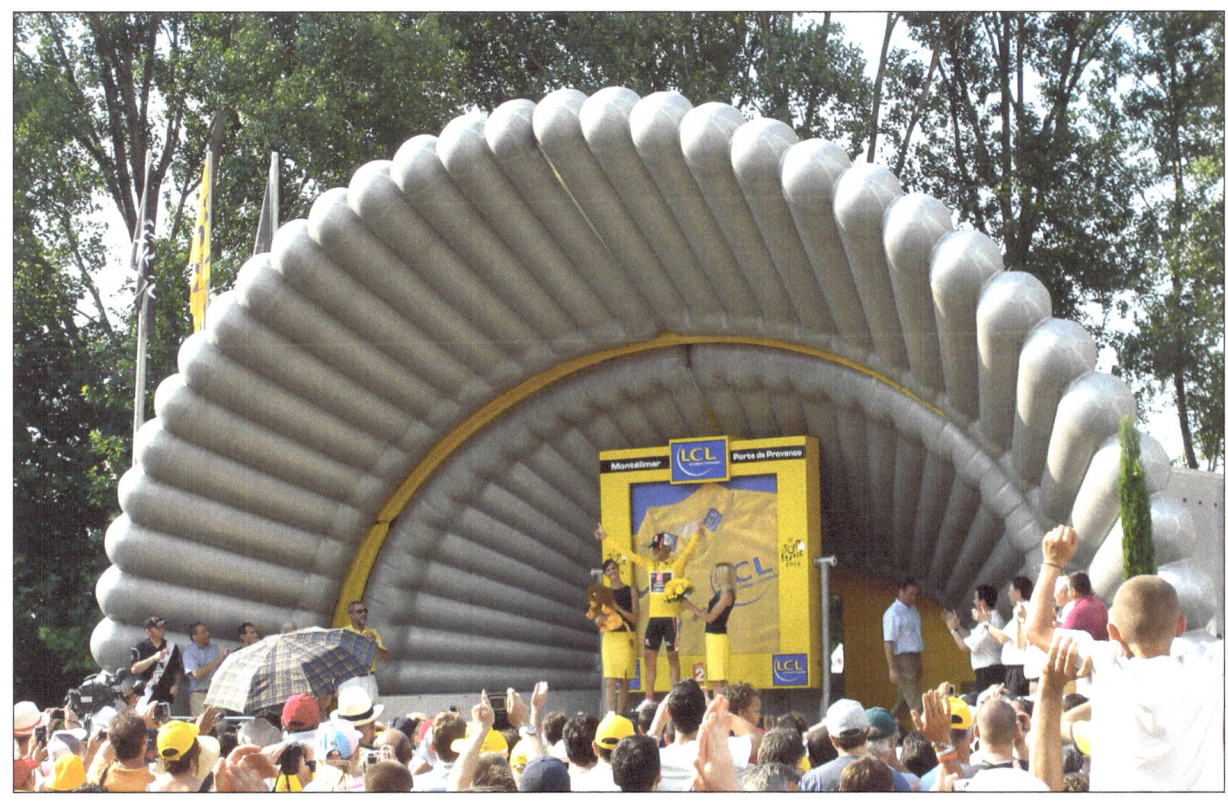

Spaniard Óscar Pereiro in the overall leader's 'Maillot Jeaune' (yellow jersey) after Stage 13 of the 2006 Tour de France, Montélimar

Le Côte d'Azur, Vence and Sanremo

Sunday, July 16th we left Malaucène and La Provençe after an exceptional, wonderful week and traveled on to Le Côte d'Azur where we would stay in Vence, another medieval village perched in the rugged, limestone hills above Antibes and Cagnes-sur-Mer. Two millennia ago it was the Roman settlement of *Vintium*,[96] built on a rocky plateau along an ancient road leading inland. The setting gave it a 'balcony' view of the Var valley and surrounding seaside. The weather felt pleasantly warm and humid. The nearby Col de Vence,[97] part of the Alpes-Maritimes, would provide an opportunity to ride and take in the view from an elevation of about a thousand meters above sea level.

Our lodgings at the *Hôtel Miramar* were perfect – another meticulously restored manor house, just a flat five minute stroll from the *Vielle Ville*.[98] We settled into the two room poolside cottage and our host Davide soon informed us that Frenchman

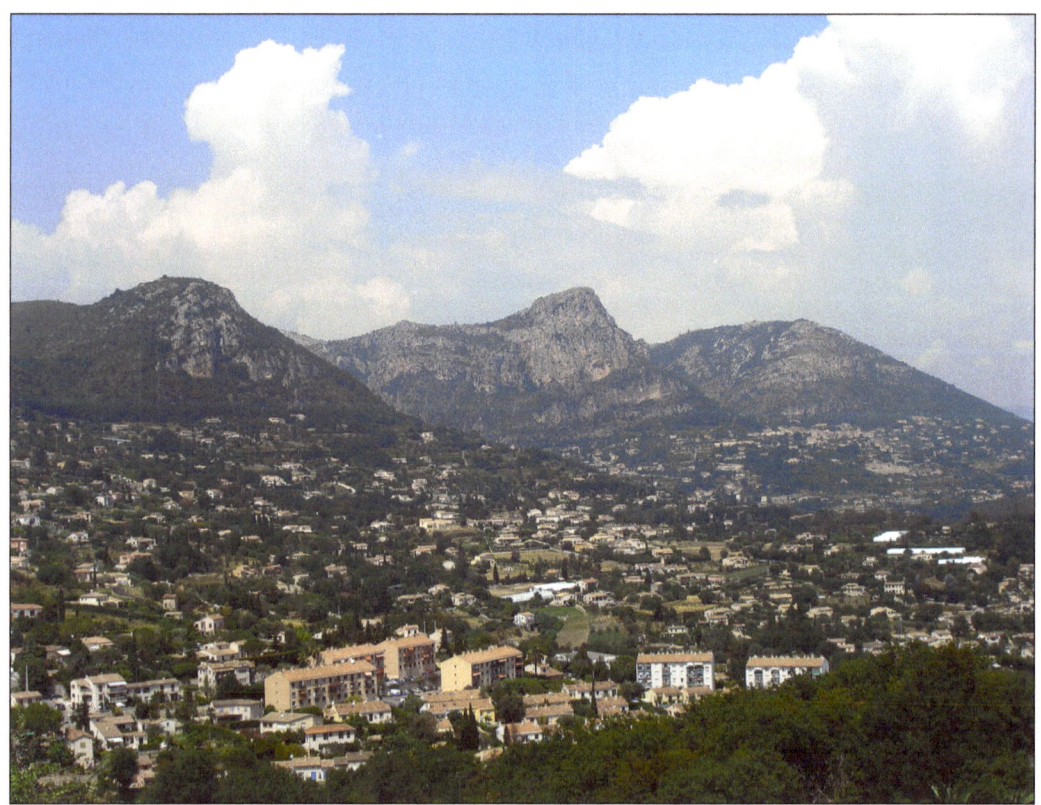

A balcony view of the Alpes-Maritimes, Vence

---

96. *Vintium* was first a colony and then a municipality after Romans claimed the Cote d'Azur.
97. The Col de Vence, elevation 963 meters (3159 feet), is a steady 5% to 7%, 10 kilometer climb through the craggy, rocky escarpments above the village.
98. The medieval city, with its intact 13th century walls.

Pierrick Fédrigo, had won the Tour's hilly 181 km Stage 14 in four hours, 14 minutes. Óscar Pereiro finished in a group just seven seconds later and kept the *maillot jeaune.* Floyd Landis stayed in 2nd place overall – one minute, 29 seconds behind Pereiro.

Monday was the Tour's second rest day. Frank and I rode to the Col de Vence and an additional seven kilometers to Coursegoules, a tiny hamlet sitting at an elevation of about 1,000 meters. The hour long ride felt similar to climbing Mount Tamalpais in Marin County, California. Bougainvillea was blooming everywhere as we left Vence and entered the *Parc Naturel Régional des Préalpes d'Azur.* There was little shade and the temperature was 86°F (30° C). The vegetation became sparse and brushy in the rocky terrain, exposing views of Vence below and the Mediterranean shore in the hazy distance. Italy was in view at the eastern horizon. The downhill return to Vence was a 'bust' as flagmen and slow moving road maintenance vehicles had appeared en masse somehow in more than one location. All in all, it was still another beautiful ride – the last of the Cols we would climb while in France.

We had a deluxe seafood dinner that evening at *Le Bistro du Peyre* in the *Vielle Ville.* It was a balmy and beautiful, perfect for an *al fresco* meal – complete with strolling musicians. The fresh mussels bisque and locally caught fish fillets with *piquante* red sauce were delicious. We enjoyed an excellent bottle of rosé and chocolate mousse for dessert. Chatting with our waitress, we learned a bit about the restaurant and asked if it might be possible to look at the wine cellar. She and the owner obliged us and the room was very *cool* – literally and figuratively. Down a stone spiral staircase we went, into a large limestone cave equipped with a piano, long table and enough chairs to seat at least twenty people. The ceiling was braced with gnarled wood and large stone blocks – the walls were heavily whitewashed. Wrought iron chandeliers hung in two places. It felt accommodating – as though many a festive banquet had taken place there!

Tuesday I celebrated my 52nd birthday – right where I wanted to be. After lunch *al fresco* near the *Hôtel de Ville,*[99] Frank and I found a nearby tavern and watched the Tour action live... and live it was! Luxembourger Frank Schleck won the tough, mountainous 187 km Stage 15, finishing on the legendary L'Alpe d'Huez in four

---

99. City Hall.

hours, 52 minutes. Having now ridden some of these high Cols, we had a true appreciation for all of the racers difficult efforts.

Floyd Landis had managed to stay with his main riders of concern in the GC and finished 4th, just one minute, 10 seconds later, taking the *maillot jeaune* from Óscar Pereiro. The Spaniard had finished 13th, another one minute, 39 seconds behind and slipped into second place in the GC, with a 10 second deficit. If Landis could keep the yellow jersey through the next two stages, he had a chance to achieve the biggest win of his career! He was expected to do well in Saturday's final time trial. Even the scandalous clouds of *Operación Puerto* couldn't dampen the intensity of the unfolding GC competition.

Wednesday we took a 'day trip' and drove east to Sanremo, across the border on the Italian Riviera. After an hour or so on the autoroute we arrived and first visited *La Pigna*,[100] an older neighborhood dating to the medieval period of the Ligurian city. I was strolling in a labyrinth of cobblestone walking streets, steep and formidable but ultimately offering grand views of the Mediterranean Sea and harbor below. Many of the 15th century houses here were constructed so closely together that the vaulted archways between them became the pedestrian alleyways of today. Churches were numerous and a strong sense of tradition came across in the bronzed faces of local people we saw congregating in the small *piazzas*.

There was no way to visit much in just an afternoon but *La Pigna* seemed as impressive as the medieval villages we had seen in France – with the added attraction of its seaside location. We passed the 100 year old *Art Nouveau style Casinò di Sanremo*,[101] San Basilio's Russian Orthodox Church and several 19th century grand hotels on our way to a small cafe near the *Porto Vecchio*.[102] There we enjoyed ice-cold *Nastro Azzurro*[103] and *Risotto di Mare* before walking to the beach where I waded into the Mediterranean for a picture. The air temperature was 100°F (approx. 38°C) – the sea felt warm, like bath water.

---

100. *La Pigna*, or 'pine cone' refers to the stair-stepped appearance of the houses built in this hilly part of the City.
101. Sanremo became popular as a holiday resort in the 18th and 19th Centuries. The Casino was built in 1905.
102. Old Port.
103. *Peroni's Nastro Azzurro* is a premium Italian pilsner beer (5.0% alcohol by volume).

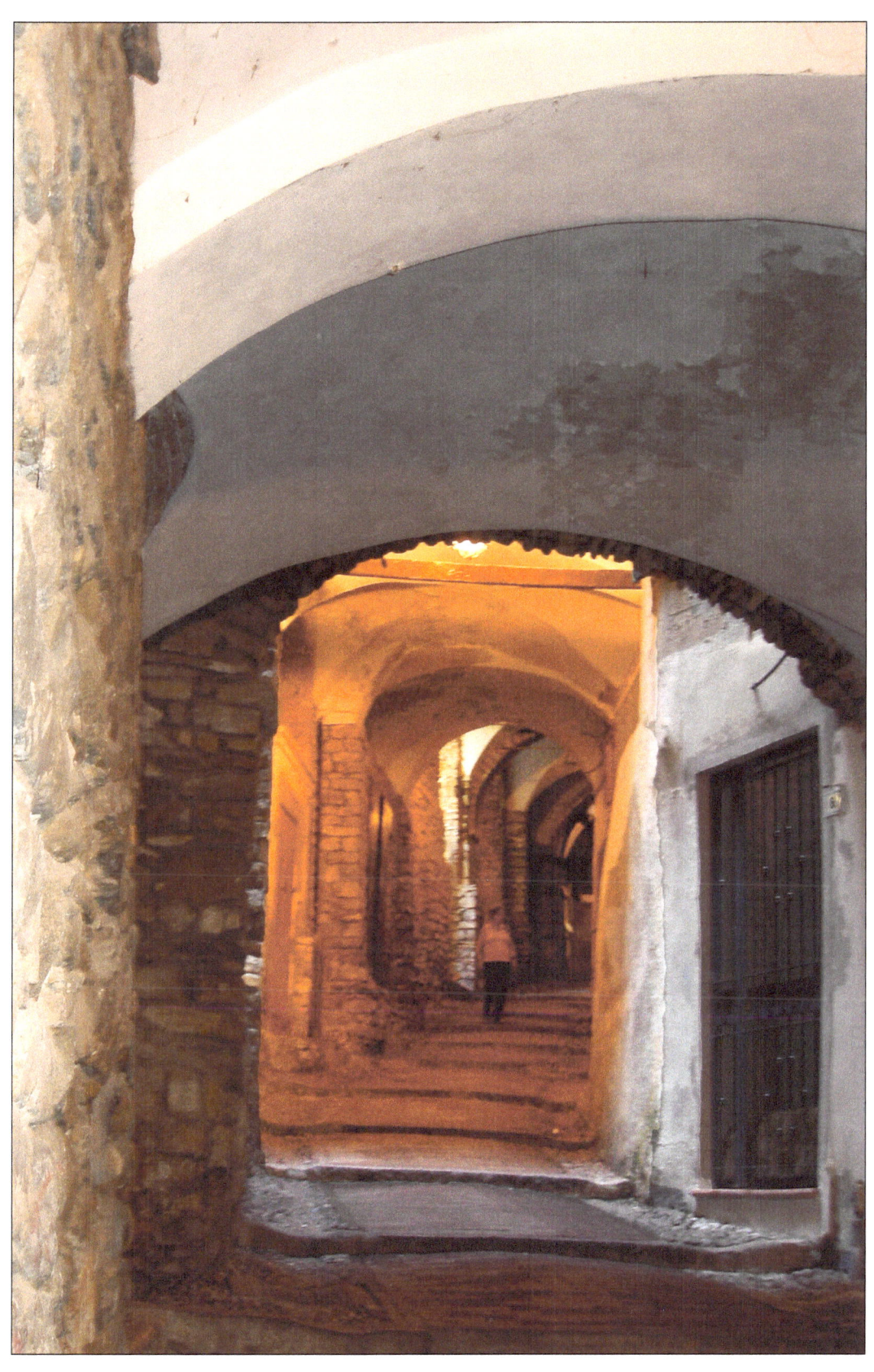

Porticato della Pigna, a covered walking street in Sanremo

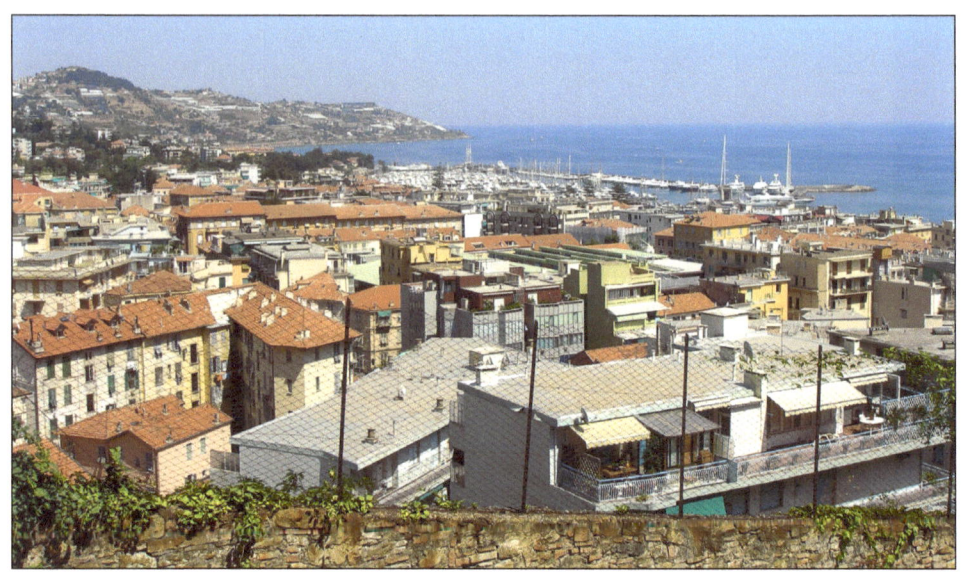

Sanremo and the 'Porto Vecchio' (old port)

While we were enjoying the late afternoon in seaside Sanremo, we had no idea that Floyd Landis was 'cracking' that day on the Stage 16's final ten km *HC* climb to La Toussuire.[104] He had begun falling behind his main rivals with 60 km left to race and finished a disastrous *eight* minutes behind Óscar Pereiro, tumbling to *11th place* in the GC. Not only had he lost the yellow jersey for the second time, he'd also seemingly blown his chances for overall victory. Had his teammate Axel Merckx[105] not been there to dutifully pace him on he would have certainly lost more time. His Tour had turned upside down. He'd *'bonked'*[106] in the *maillot jeaune* – on the world stage!

Landis' Tour seemed ruined but Denmark's Michael Rasmussen's had gotten better. He had raced away from the peloton and ridden solo for *70 km*, winning the mountainous 182 km Stage 16, in five hours, 36 minutes. He would go on to win the overall Polka Dot jersey competition.[107] Óscar Pereiro finished 3rd, one minute, 54 seconds behind the Dane, retaking

---

104. 18 km climb at 6.1%, reaching an elevation of 1694 meters.
105. The Belgian racer (now retired) is the son of the legendary Eddy Merckx.
106. 'Bonking' is cycling jargon for the experience of being suddenly depleted of the energy needed to continue riding at a pace above minimum. Symptoms can typically include temporarily losing the ability to use one's leg strength, the inability to keep pedaling a constant cadence and a feeling of heaviness in the legs. Bonking can often take place while climbing a hill, thus the phrase 'hitting the wall' has become synonymous.
107. General Classification - Yellow Jersey, Points Classification - Green Jersey, Mountain Classification - Polka Dot Jersey, Best Young Rider Classification - White Jersey

the *maillot jeaune*. Merckx and Landis rolled over the finish line in 22nd and 23rd place, just over ten minutes after Rasmussen. Landis bolted to a team car and quickly left the race venue, avoiding the swarm of reporters and photographers. He appeared strangely calm and circumspect when he was interviewed later at his team's hotel. It had been a disastrous day for him and he seemed to smile as he explained having a "very bad day on the wrong day." He no longer expected to win.

Frank and I were now fully committed to following the Tour's *live* broadcast. Of course, there was a 'rush to judgement' by so many about what had happened and whether Landis could recover enough to get back in the race. Former Tour champions had already called this year's tour *bizarre* – picking the 2006 race winner had now become almost anyone's guess. Less than three minutes separated the top five leaders with only three days of racing left. Thursday would be the last difficult Alpine stage. The drama was palpable. We opted to hang out by the Hotel Miramar's pool and follow the race action live. It was the perfect choice – the mountainous 200 km Stage 17 proved to be the most exciting of all!

Spaniard Carlos Sastre, German Andreas Klöden and the other contenders rode strong on the tough Stage 17 but Floyd Landis was on a mission. The American – described as having 'no panache' – now had nothing to lose. His team pressed the pace at the front of the peloton early on and Landis then pulled away – just a quarter of the way into the race. With a fast steady effort he caught and passed the day's breakaway riders, eventually gaining over *eight* minutes on the chasing group before the final climb, an ascent of the Col de Joux-Plane.[108] He won the stage solo – in an incredible five hours, 24 minutes! Floyd Landis crossed the finish with a fist pump and no smile... his gamble had paid off. The French press called it *La Chevauchée Fantastique.*[109]

Óscar Pereiro was down the mountain and finished with the main chasers, just over seven minutes behind. Pereiro remained in the *maillot jeaune* but after an incredible day of redemption,

---

108. An 11.6 km climb at 8.6%, reaching an elevation of 1,689 meters, 25 km from the finish.
109. The Fantastic Ride. In medieval warfare, *la chevauchée* referred to a rapid horse charge attack.

Landis had regained his position as a contender for the overall victory. Amazingly, his deficit was now just 30 seconds! Stage 18 was destined to be critical as they would leave the mountains. It was also clear that Saturday's final time trial would be decisive for the GC. Frank and I were fine with that – we already planned to be there, watching from somewhere on the course.

Stage 17 had included the most exciting finish in years – but something felt strange again. After an amazing victory Floyd Landis had appeared *angry* at the finish line. He was smiling later on as he discussed his chances for the overall win but the questions were unavoidable. How was such a comeback possible? Was it something physical? Had the peloton let him ride away? All through the month there had been the odorous background of *Operación Puerto* and now the rumors and suspicions had become more focused on him. The Tour's directors were reaffirming their continuing fight against doping and the media began having a field day, with speculation and doubts that someone 'clean' could accomplish such a victory – a single day after faltering so dramatically. The current doping scandal and the era of allegations against Lance Armstrong had tainted the Tour. It was obvious that many fans felt it might be a case of *'Here we go again'* with Landis, his former teammate.

After watching the Tour coverage and hearing Floyd Landis speak, Frank and I were excited but both thinking *'I sure hope it ain't so'* as opposed to *'Here we go again'* regarding his day's race results. It was pretty clear that Floyd Landis would have some explaining to do in his near future. We made the short walk from our hotel to the *Vielle Ville* for one last fine dinner in Vence – at *La Litote*. No surprise – it was predictably superb and a much needed distraction from the race. The strolling guitar trio played while we ate on the terrace. My seafood tasted the best yet – *Saumon Roti et fondant*[110] with summer vegetables and a *Salade de Chevre aux graines de pivot bleu*. A crisp rosé with the meal followed by Napoleon brandy and *sorbet au citron* for dessert made it memorable.

---

110. In a white wine sauce.

Gueugnon, the final Time Trial and Paris-Redux

Friday, July 21st we left Vence and began our travel back to Paris – first returning to the south of Burgundy where the Tour's final time trial would take place the following day. Frank and I had plenty of time to talk about the previous day's astounding, confusing comeback by Floyd Landis. His chances for winning the Tour had exploded and re-materialized in two days! He and Óscar Pereiro had exchanged the leader's jersey three times now – it wasn't getting any easier to pick a winner. The 2006 Tour had been a tough race, made even tougher by the backdrop of *Operación Puerto's* activities and revelations about doping. After heading north through Valence and Lyon to Mâcon, we followed departmental roads to Gueugnon, situated on a tributary of the Loire River. The temperatures here were the hottest we'd seen – reaching 108°F (42°C).

Rather than explore the village we opted for *hors d'ourves* in our hotel's air-conditioned bar while quenching our thirst with *Kronenbourg* and watching the Tour's news and a rebroadcast of the day's race. Italian Matteo Tossato had won the rolling 197 km Stage 18, sprinting to victory in four hours, 16 minutes. Óscar Pereiro's group finished eight minutes behind but he was to keep the *maillot jeaune* for a fifth day. Floyd Landis was still with him, thirty seconds behind – sitting in 3rd place, overall. It was a strategy that favored Landis' chances of gaining time the following day.

Saturday morning we headed to Montceau-les-Mines to watch the Tour's decisive Stage 19 final time trial. We walked to a turn along the course ideal for photos, shade and proximity to concessionaires selling cold drinks. The air felt dry and it was easily 104°F (40°C). Approximately 1:30 pm, the first riders began to roll through. Our position was just 10 kilometers from the finish and quite a few racers were catching their *two minute* man.[111]

In an individual time trial the participants are racing alone – against the clock. I managed to get close up images of the leading racers rolling by, followed by a team car displaying their name on the front of the vehicle. Despite the heat, Sergei Honchar

---

111. Racers often start at two minute intervals in a time trial event.

won the flat 57 km stage 19 in one hour, seven minutes, 45 seconds but most importantly, Floyd Landis achieved his goal! He finished third, just one minute, 11 seconds later, regaining the *maillot jeaune* and effectively *winning* the 2006 Tour! He had bested Óscar Pereiro's 4th place time by one minute, 29 seconds and now held a 59 second advantage. Landis and Pereiro had exchanged the *maillot jeaune* for a *fourth* and last time!

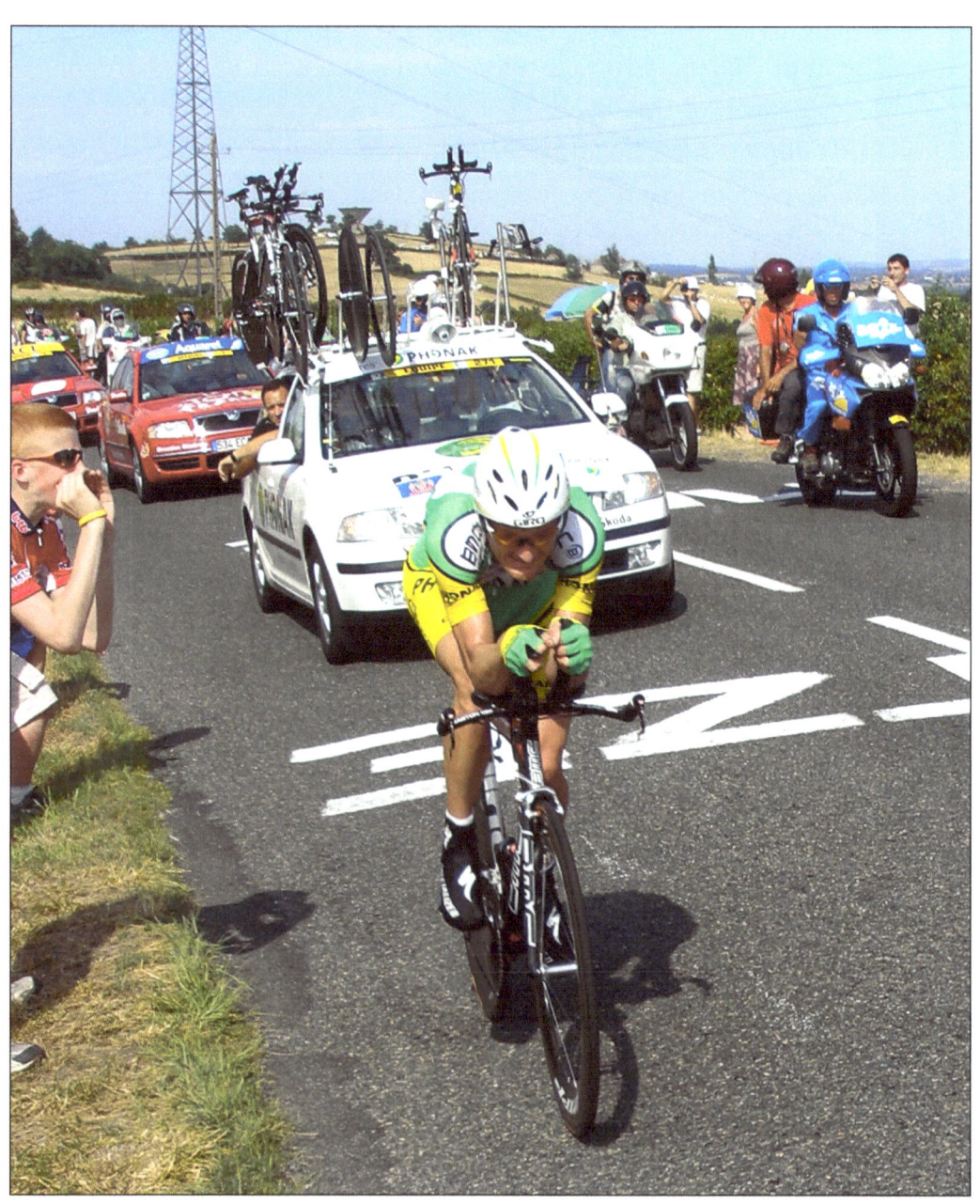

Floyd Landis racing against the clock towards his 'win' in the 2006 Tour de France, Montceau-les-Mines

There was an unceremonious feeling of anticlimax that day – effectively the finish of the 2006 Tour. *Operación Puerto* had been a persistent cloud for the entire three weeks and the puzzling performance and surprise comeback victory by Floyd Landis had also raised obvious questions, dampening the sense of jubilation. Something about the win felt sinister and many racers and fans were clearly uncomfortable with the results. Pro cycling was facing the undeniable truth that nine racers had been removed from this year's Tour before it began and an impending revelation would soon bookend the race with more scandal.

After the race we followed departmental roads to the autoroute. A steady downpour made it a slow drive and we arrived in Paris about 10:30 pm. The rain had stopped and for the third time, the exact same parking place in front of our apartment was vacant! After unloading our gear we stepped out to have a 'nightcap,' smoke a *Cubano* and celebrate our successful return to Paris. Later at the apartment we watched the news coverage of the controversial Tour's final competitive race day.

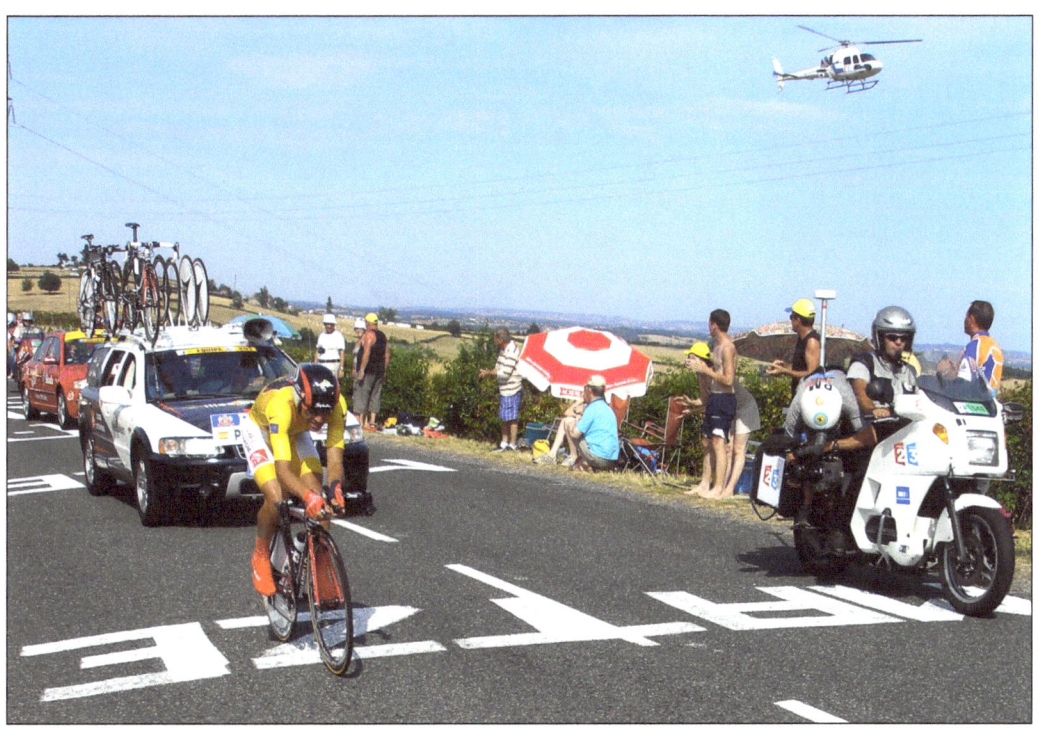

Óscar Pereiro at Montceau-les-Mines, losing time to Floyd Landis

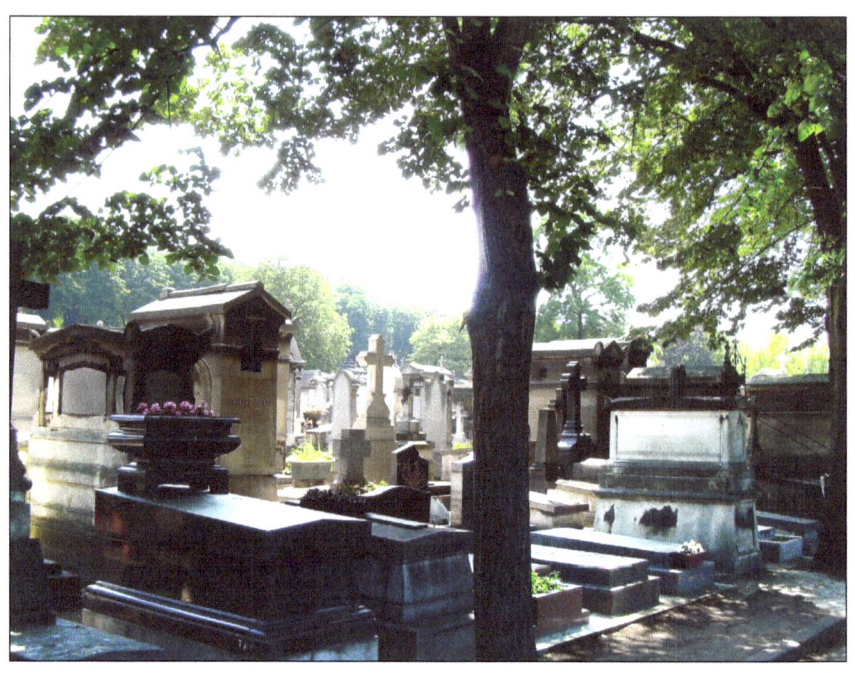

Père Lachaise Cimitière, Paris

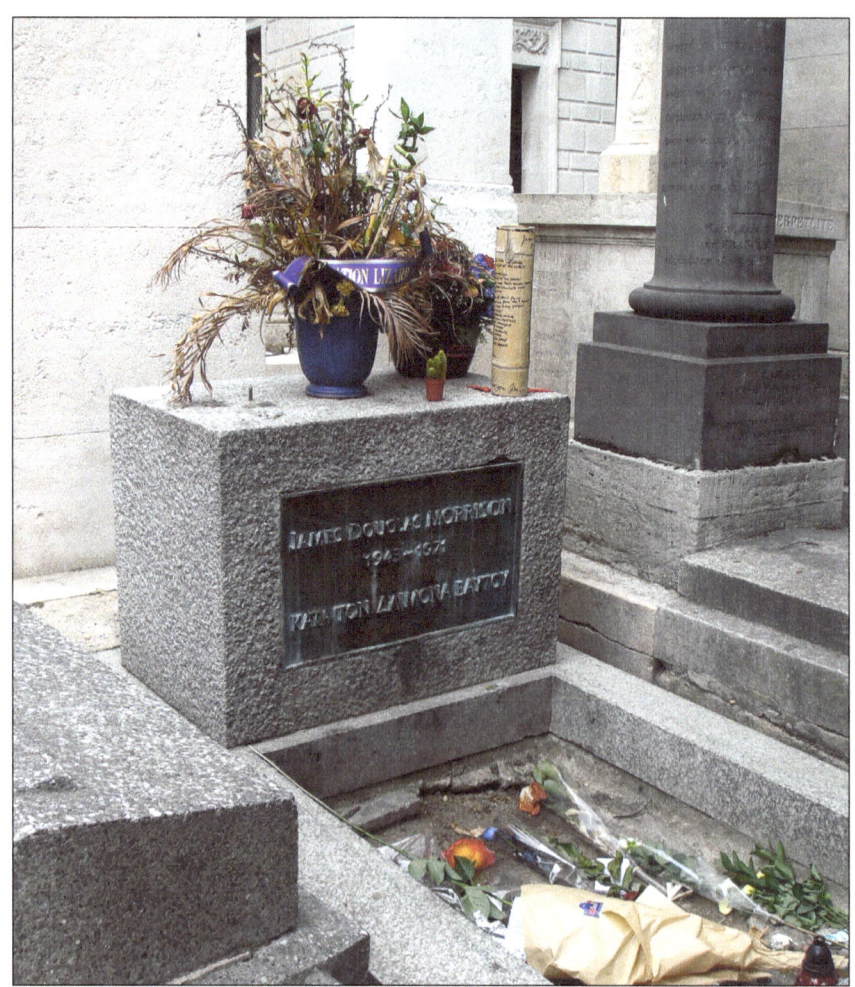

Jim Morrison's grave in Père Lachaise Cimitière, Paris

Sunday morning we returned the rental car and then walked to the venerable Cimitière du Père Lachaise to look for Jim Morrison's grave before heading to the Tour's finale near the Place de la Concorde. It was slightly morbid but obligatory for me, having grown up near San Francisco during the 'hippie days' of the 1960s listening to the music of *The Doors* and other west coast rock musicians. His frequently visited gravesite is surprisingly simple and modest – even obscure, among the many elaborate and impressive monuments placed there for other famous people.

From Père Lachaise we strolled along the *quais* at the River Seine, passing the *Paris Riviera,* where a manmade 'sandy beach' is constructed annually. Hundreds of people were out relaxing, seemingly oblivious to the *Tour de France*, sunbathing and entertaining themselves as if they were at the seaside.

Around noon we made our way to the Champs Élysées where the arrival of the Tour's racers en masse prompted mostly cheers from the huge crowds. After failing in our attempts to position ourselves anywhere near the finish line, we settled for an area along the Quai des Tuileries which turned out to be perfect. I captured images of the teams riding together during the later part of the race.

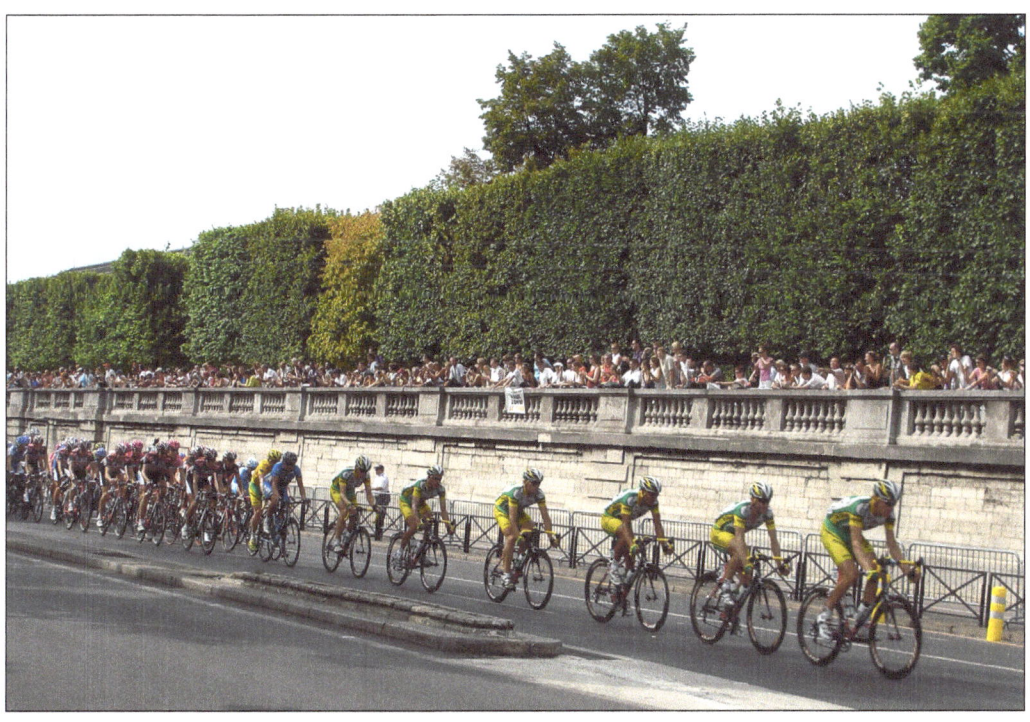

Team Phonak leading Floyd Landis (8th position) along the Quai des Tuileries, Paris

After eight laps of the traditional circuit between the Arc d'Triomphe and the Place de la Concorde, Thor Hushovd won the large bunch sprint for the mostly flat 155 km Stage 20, finishing in just under three hours, 57 minutes. For the General Classification it was a ceremonial conclusion. Floyd Landis crossed the Champs Élysées holding a 57 second lead over Óscar Periero and was declared the winner – at least temporarily. The podium ceremony was held. Media reactions ranged from amazement to condemnation.

Monday I packed my bike for the trip home and took it easy. In the evening Frank and I walked to the Place de Vosges where we had one last, fine French meal at *Ma Bourgogne.* Dinner was as expected, excellent *and* expensive – filet mignon with mushrooms, potatoes and shallots, Bordeaux red wine, a salad with goat cheese and shredded carrots, all followed by *crème brûlée* fit for a dessert connoisseur.

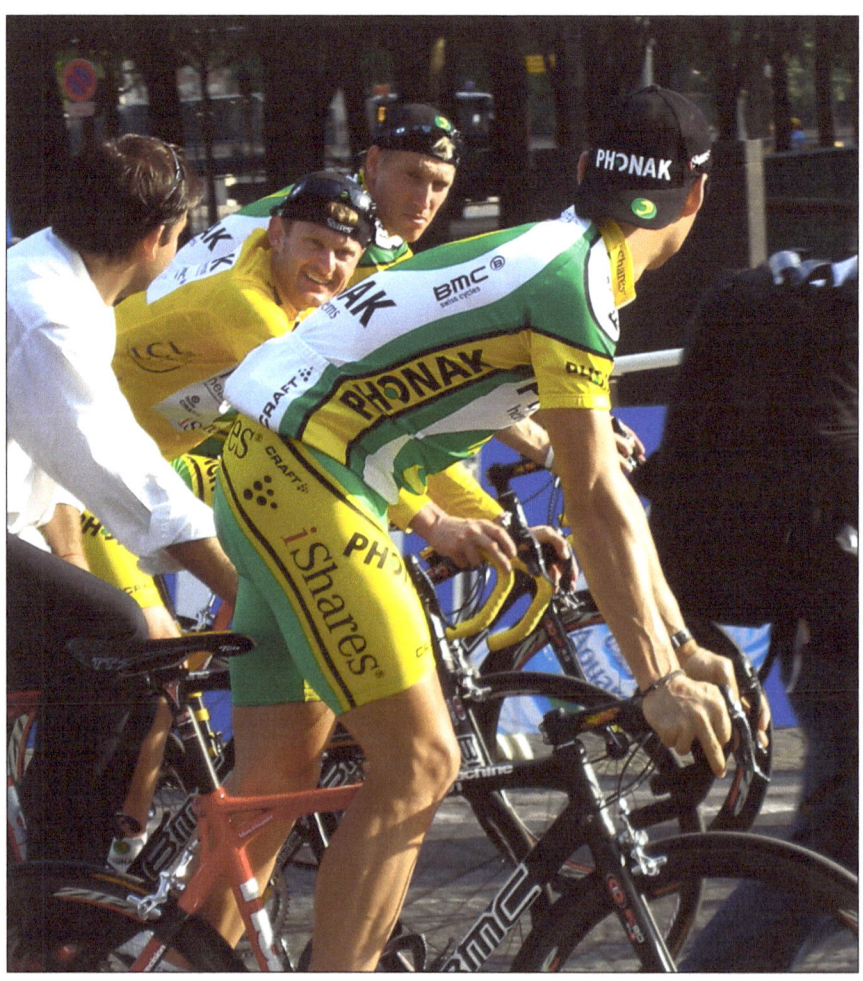

Floyd Landis celebrates a 'victory' lap with team mates Alexandre Moos (f) and Axel Mercks (r) on the Place de la Concorde

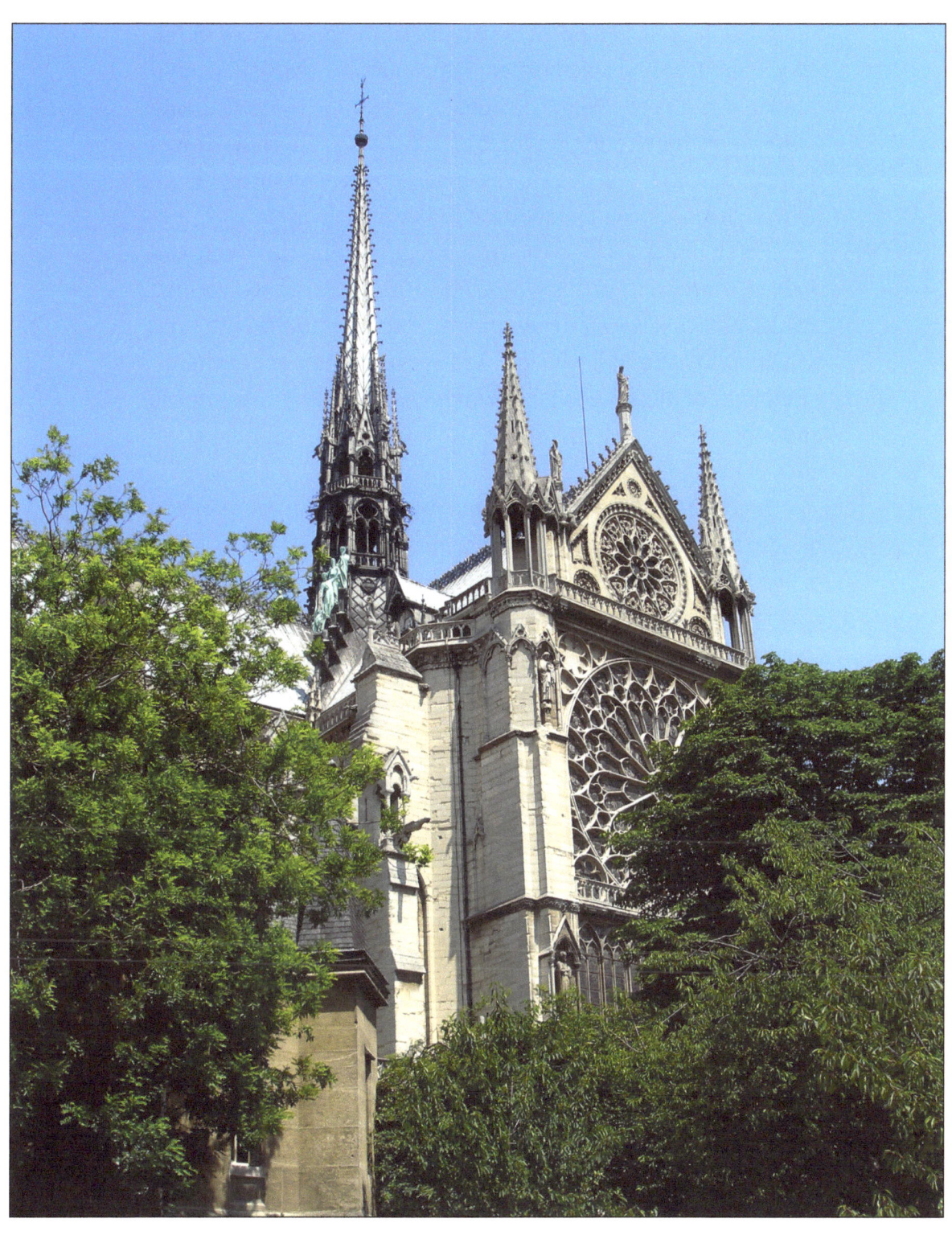

**Rose windows and Gothic spires of the mid 13th century
Cathédrale Notre-Dame de Paris**

Tuesday, July 25th was my last full day in France. I packed and tried to read *L'Equipe*. The wolves of the press were in full attack mode as suspicions and speculation swirled around Landis – his remarkable comeback and victory were being widely questioned and the worst for him was yet to come. It was difficult to watch him put 'on the spot' in television interviews – he was clearly uncomfortable and evasive.

Frank and I decided to stroll along the Rue du Rivoli and walked to the *Cathédrale Notre Dame de Paris* where we had drinks at the nearby *Café Quasimodo*. I ducked into the Cathedral which was tremendous inside. As I sat for a moment in the filtered light of the stained glass windows the feeling was intense and immediate – a sense of historic events and longtime presence of human spirit there was undeniable.

A group tour began, disrupting my contemplation. I walked back to the Café and Frank and I decided to have *two* last drinks – to our amazing journey *and* an easy trip home. Nearby, an old man played guitar while a young woman sang. Fire eaters and sword swallowers performed nearby behind them. Across the crowded plaza the monumental bronze statue of Charlemagne and his Guards[112] stood silently above all. The Cathedral bells tolled – a perfect moment, capping up a truly unique experience – a month of unforgettable adventures in France. I was looking forward to returning home but it surely had been *'Mission: Accomplished'*... my own remarkable *Tour de France*, both on and off the bike!

---

112. Charlemagne et ses Leudes, or Charlemagne and his Guards, by Louis and Charles Rochet, 1878.

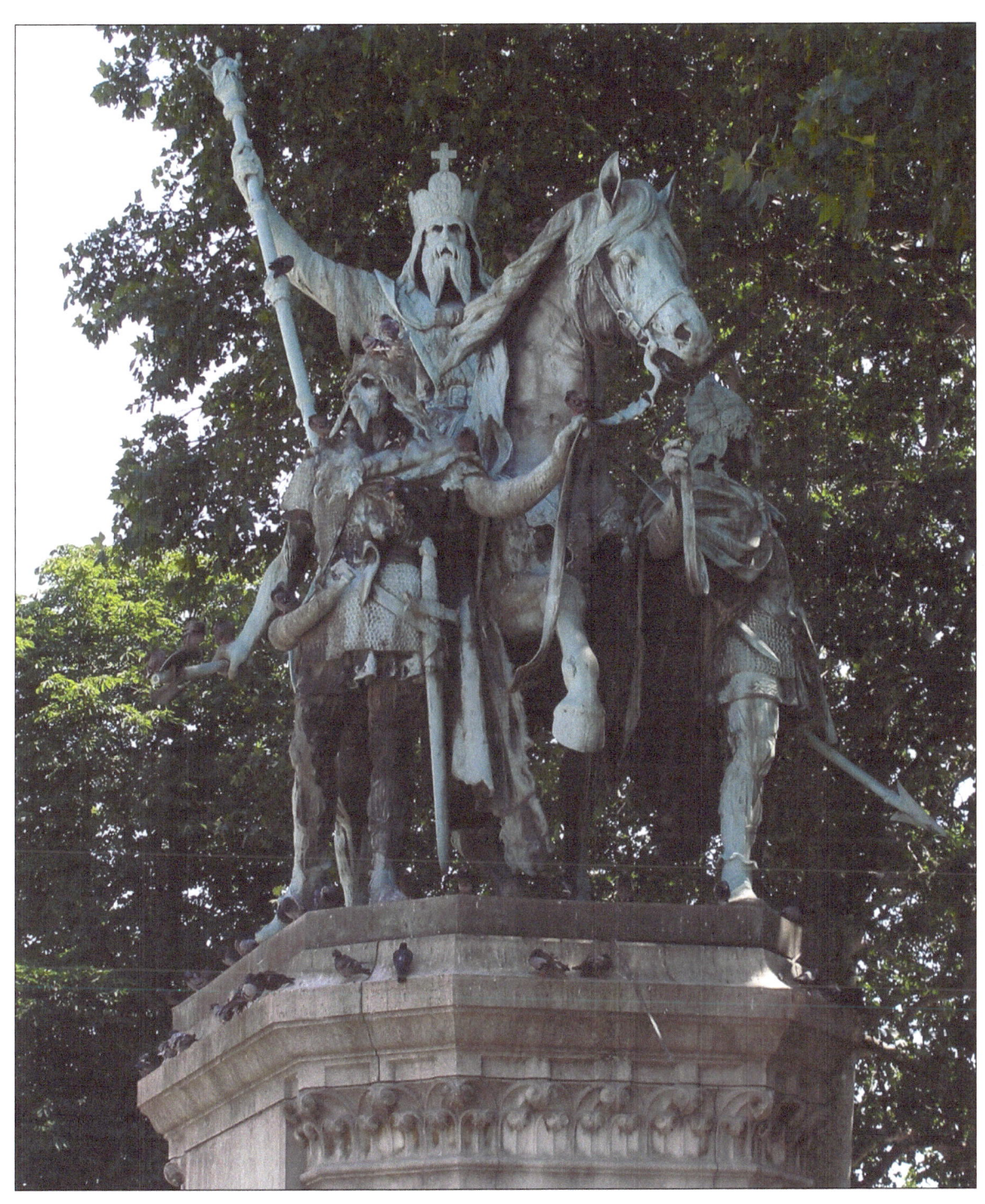

Charlemagne et ses Leudes, Louis and Charles Rochet, 1878

Getting Home and...

Wednesday morning, July 26th I departed Paris on my return flight to San Francisco. Passengers boarded the plane on time but were only en route after a *two* hour delay on the tarmac! It was an Airbus carrying several hundred diverse people, the vast majority not speaking French *or* English. It seemed quite strange but I distracted myself by trying to read the latest *L'Equipe*. Rumors were now spreading that one of the racers had returned an abnormal test result on a Stage 17 urine sample. Something in my head told me that what should have been the most exciting Tour de France in years was about to unravel.

As we flew over the Arctic, the vast expanse of melting sea ice looked like a visual metaphor for the 2006 Tour – countless, small icebergs were drifting and disintegrating into a cold slush where there should have been solid pack ice! Roughly ten hours later the crew received a rousing ovation from passengers when we had landed safely at San Francisco.

It was still July 26th here in the USA when the UCI announced that the race winner had failed a drug test. The story then exploded and Team Phonak[113] confirmed that it was their rider – the 'winner' – Floyd Landis! I wasn't really surprised – he had tested positive for synthetic testosterone, having three times the allowable ratio of testosterone to epitestosterone![114] Of course, Landis initially denied it... He played the part of a mystified victim but came across more like a child explaining to his teacher that a dog ate his homework. Nevertheless, he withdrew from the Chaarm Criterium, his next scheduled race in the Netherlands. As *L'Equipe* put it, there was *un air de déjà vu!*

A week later Landis' 'B' sample had also returned a positive, confirming his earlier results and sealing his fate – he would become the first disqualified 'winner' of the *Tour de France* in over 100 years.[115] The race directors no longer considered him

---

113. Floyd Landis was the lead rider for the Swiss-based, Phonak team, sponsored by Phonak Hearing Systems.
114. A maximum ratio of 4:1 is allowed. Floyd Landis test results were 12:1. Eventually, it was determined that Landis failed four of the six drug tests made on urine samples from his 2006 Tour de France.
115. The first Tour de France winner disqualification occurred in 1904, when Maurice Garin was stripped of his *1904* victory and banned for two years, after 'taking a train' instead of riding his bike on a portion of the course.

the 2006 victor. He was fired by Team Phonak immediately and the team itself disbanded ten days later. No matter how much Landis claimed he was being victimized by the labs and "French based, anti American press" it was difficult to feel sorry for him. He had damaged the credibility of a sport already marred by deep cynicism. The scandal began affecting the popularity of cycling in the USA immediately. Fallout from his hypocrisy and arrogance would impact the professional peloton from top to bottom – for years. The Tour was mocked in headlines reading 'Le Tour de Fraud' and 'Le Tour de Dope.'

The Tour was marooned somewhere in a sea of lies but, as is often the case, at some point the truth *emerges*. Perhaps the scandal's aftermath was predictable – after years of claiming innocence amidst numerous investigations and arbitration, Floyd Landis admitted doping through most of his career in May of 2010. He also 'blew the whistle' on other American riders[116] who would eventually receive suspensions and lose their race results for the 2006 tour. Lance Armstrong would be implicated as well and famously admit to systematic doping on the US Postal Service team in 2013. Armstrong was stripped of all seven of his *Tour de France* 'victories' in August of 2012.[117]

Why did it matter? Well, it seemed that the wheels of change began turning in July of 2006. Ultimately, Stage 17 had huge consequences and started a period that continues to influence all professional riders today. Along with all of the other 'once in a lifetime' experiences Frank and I had those five weeks, we unintentionally witnessed the beginning of the end of systematic industrial-scale doping programs in our beloved sport of bicycle racing. It took a while to hold the guilty accountable but the current generation of racers has reaped the benefits of a modern era where 'doping is cheating.' As a wise man once said "no doubt the universe is unfolding as it should."[118]

---

116. George Hincapie, Levi Leipheimer and David Zabriskie would also admit to doping,
117. There is no official Tour de France winner for the years: 1999-2005.
118. Max Ehrmann, from his piece *Desiderata*, 1927.

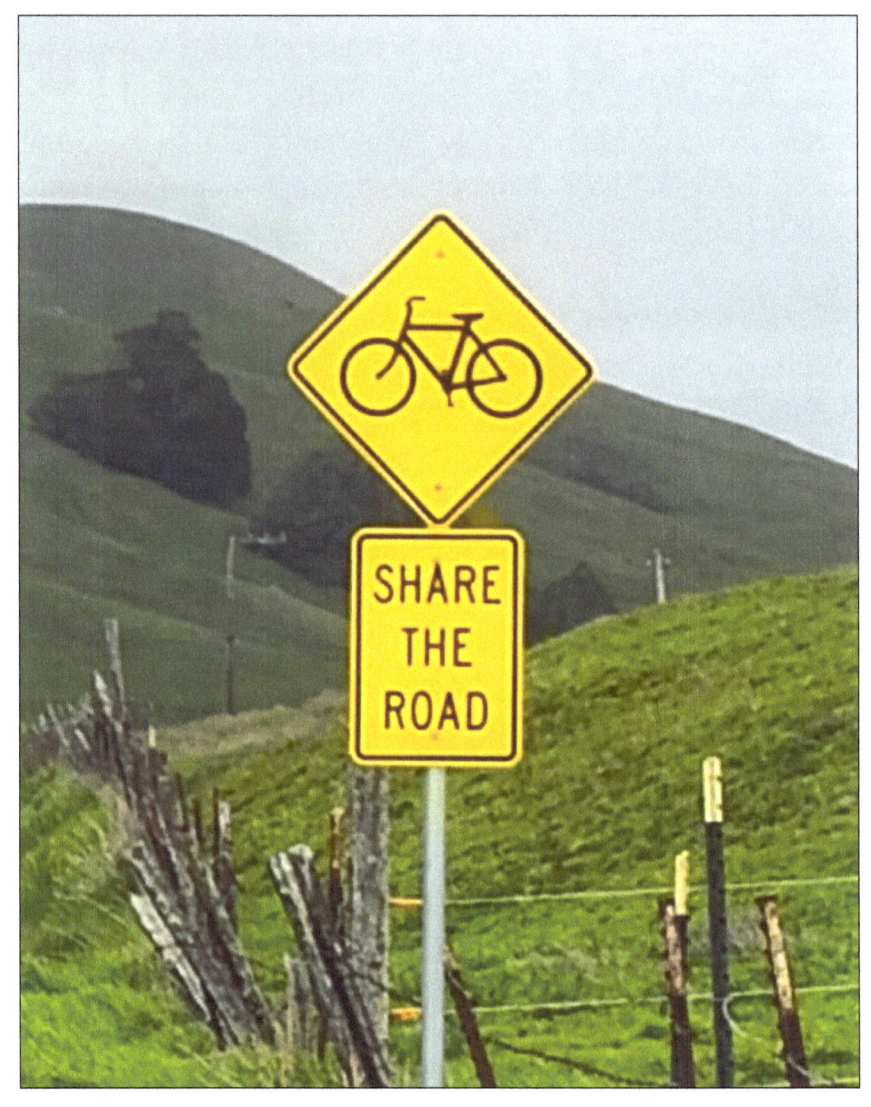

Index of Selected Places

Agoura 44
Alameda 84
Alamo 89
Albany 6
Algona 118
Alpes-Maritimes 138, 182
Anthueil 153
Antibes 182
Ashford 109

Barbizon 143
Beaume de Venise 175
Beaune 152
Berkeley 78
Besse-en-Oisans 157
Bibracte 157
Blackhawk 89
Briançon 167
Bourg d'Oisans 157
Buckley 109

Cagnes-sur-Mer 182
Carpinteria 43
Carson 56
Castle Rock 121
Cayucos 34
Centerville 65
Centralia 120
Chablis 151
Chaux 155
Chehalis 120
Clavans-en-Haute-Oisans 160
Clayton 88
Concord 88
Contra Costa County 3, 86
Corvallis 117
Côte-d'Or 150
Coursegoules 183

Daly City 132
Dentelles de Montmirail 175
Double Spring Flat 65

Eatonville 109
El Cerrito 75
El Toro 53
Elbe 109
Enumclaw 106

Fontainebleau 138, 141
France 137

Gap 167
Gaviota 39
Gigondas 175
Goble 122
Goleta 42
Gordes 178
Greenwater 111
Grenoble 157
Guadalupe 36
Gueugnon 189

Hercules 86
Huntington Beach 53

Kathmandu 92
Kelso 121
Kent 118

L'Alpe d'Huez 157, 161
L'République 141
La Bourgogne 138, 150
La Provence 138, 167
Lafare 175
Lafayette 90
Lake Tahoe 31, 58, 83
Las Cruces 40
Le Côte d'Azur 138, 182
Lindbergh 122
Livermore 88
Lompoc 35
Longmire 109
Longview 121
Los Angeles 29, 33

Malibu 49
Marin County 15, 21, 59
Markleeville 60
Malaucène 169
Meyers 62
Mill Valley 21, 83
Milly-la Forêt 143, 146
Mission Viejo 53
Mont Ventoux 172
Montceau-les-Mines 189
Montecito 43
Montigny-la-Resle 150
Montélimar 180
Morro Bay 35
Muir Beach 16, 21
Murs 178

Napavine 120
Newport Bay 53
Nisqually 106
Nuits-St. George 155
Nyon 169

Ocean Park 38
Oceano 36
Orting 109
Oxnard 44

Pacific 118
Pantoll Station 16, 22
Paradise 106
Paris 138, 141, 189
Paso Robles 34
Pinole 3, 7, 90
Pismo Beach 36
Pleasant Hill 88
Point Mugu 49
Point Reyes Station 16
Port Hueneme 44
Portland 113
Puyallup 113

Rainier 122
Redmond 116
Renton 118
Rhône-Alpes 138, 157
Roy 118

St. Jean de Maurienne 163
St. Michel de Maurienne 163
San Francisco 29, 34, 117, 139
San Francisco Bay 15, 21, 128
San Lorenzo 85, 137
San Luis Obispo County 34
San Romain 153
Sanremo 182
Santa Barbara 38, 43
Santa Monica 15
Sausalito 15, 21, 29
Savigny-lès-Beaune 153
Scappoose 122
Seattle 105, 113
South Lake Tahoe 59
Spanaway 118
St. Helens 122
Stateline 68
Stinson Beach 16, 21
Strasbourg 148
Summerland 43
Sumner 118
Suzette 175

Tamalpais Valley Junction 23
Tara Hills 10
Tenino 119

Vader 120
Vaisson-la-Romaine 175
Vacqueyras 175
Valence 189
Vasio Vocontiorum 176
Venasque 178
Vence 182
Ventura 39, 44, 49
Verclause 168
Villers-la-Faye 155
Vintium 182

Walnut Creek 90
Westlake Village 45
Winlock 120
Woodfords 65

Yelm 118
Yreka 117

Acknowledgements

Maps, profiles and other graphics by Jonathan Van Coops.

A world of thanks and love to Alina Smiotanko, for her constant supportive energy, patience and participation in everything from field work to photography.

Many thanks to Thomas H. Mikkelsen and Frank Varvaro for their photography, review and their enthusiasm for this project. Some of my best cycling adventures took place with these two fellow cyclists 'along for the ride.' A high degree of familiarity with the ride and story details made their input invaluable.

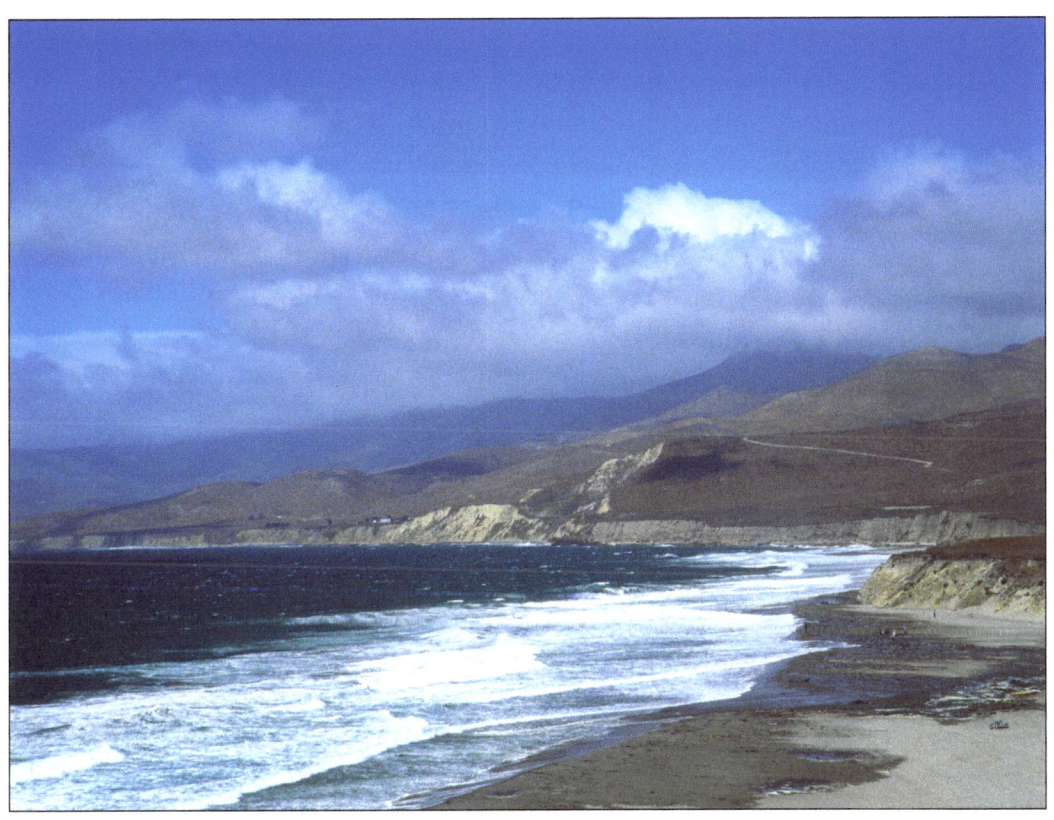

Jalama Beach, western Santa Barbara County

About the Author

Jonathan Van Coops was one of those kids to whom a bicycle gave wings. He grew up in the 1960s riding the city streets of San Francisco area's East Bay flatlands. By 1970, he had nailed cleats on to his cycling shoes and began riding his modest French ten-speed road bike gradually further into the hilly Regional Parks and watershed lands east of Berkeley.

A lover of bike racing but not a licensed racer himself, he became a decent climber by necessity and began focusing on longer distance rides in his teens and twenties. Three and four-hour rides covering 60 miles or more became regular weekend workouts. Throughout his thirties and forties he rode constantly and completed the various San Francisco area 'century' rides and an array of west coast long-distance cycling events.

After many miles on the trusty *Peugeot*, he began assembling a varied collection of bikes in the 1980s. At one point, he owned steel-framed and *Campagnolo*-equipped *Colnago*, *Masi* and *Coppi* road racers, a *Schwinn* Paramount track bike, *Santana* tandem, and a pre-WWII *Schwinn* balloon-tire cruiser complete with 'tanks' and horn. Since 2006, he's ridden another steel road bike, this frame custom-designed and crafted by East Bay master builder, Bernie Mikkelsen.

Repeated hip, shoulder and wrist surgeries during the past forty years have definitely impacted his current cycling adventures. His regular routes have become shorter and flatter but he continues to ride almost daily. Now at 70, his jaunts on the 'Red Mikk' are typically in the one or two hour range, leaving plenty of time for his other passions: cartography, writing and a growing group of granddaughters.

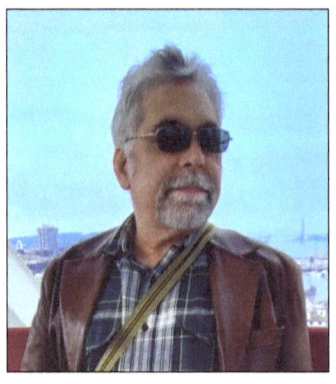

www.ingramcontent.com/pod-product-compliance
Lightning Source LLC
Chambersburg PA
CBHW041528070526
44586CB00002B/10